W9-CRN-353

DIGITAL

MEDICINE

Implications for

Healthcare Leaders

American College of Healthcare Executives
Management Series Editorial Board

Ralph H. Clark, Jr., FACHE
Eastern Health System, Inc., Birmingham, AL

Terence T. Cunningham, III, FACHE
Ben Taub General Hospital, Houston, TX

Carolyn C. Carpenter, CHE
Duke University Hospital, Durham, NC

Marie de Martinez, FACHE
St. Francis Medical Center, Grand Island, NE

Sandra A. DiPasquale, Dr.P.H., FACHE
Community Health Center of Buffalo, Inc., Buffalo, NY

Irene Fleshner, CHE
Genesis Health Ventures, Kennett Square, PA

Alan O. Freeman, FACHE
Big Springs Medical Association, Ellington, MO

James L. Goodloe, FACHE
Tennessee Hospital Association, Nashville, TN

MAJ Michael S. Heimall, CHE
Office of the Surgeon General, United States Army, Falls Church, VA

Kathryn S. Maginnis, CHE
Department of Veterans Affairs, Washington, DC

Gerald J. Maier, FACHE
OU Medical Center, Oklahoma City, OK

Warren K. West, CHE
Copley Hospital, Morrisville, VT

Alan M. Zuckerman, FACHE
Health Strategies/Solutions, Philadelphia, PA

DIGITAL MEDICINE

Implications for

Healthcare Leaders

Jeff Goldsmith, Ph.D.

Health Administration Press

ACHE Management Series

Your board, staff, or clients may also benefit from this book's insight. For more information on quantity discounts, contact the Health Administration Press Marketing Manager at (312) 424-9470.

This publication is intended to provide accurate and authoritative information in regard to the subject matter covered. It is sold, or otherwise provided, with the understanding that the publisher is not engaged in rendering professional services. If professional advice or other expert assistance is required, the services of a competent professional should be sought.

The statements and opinions contained in this book are strictly those of the author(s) and do not represent the official positions of the American College of Healthcare Executives, of the Foundation of the American College of Healthcare Executives, or of the Association of University Programs in Health Administration.

Copyright © 2003 by the Foundation of the American College of Healthcare Executives. Printed in the United States of America. All rights reserved. This book or parts thereof may not be reproduced in any form without written permission of the publisher.

07   06   05   04   03   5   4   3   2   1

Library of Congress Cataloging-in-Publication Data

Goldsmith, Jeff Charles.
    Digital medicine : implications for healthcare leaders / Jeff Goldsmith.
      p. cm.
    Includes bibliographical references.
    ISBN 1-56793-211-8 (alk. paper)
      1. Medical informatics. I. Title.
    R858.G656 2003
    610'.285—dc21

                                                                     2003047810

The paper used in this publication meets the minimum requirements of American National Standard for Information Sciences—Permanence of Paper for Printed Library Materials, ANSI Z39.48-1984. ⊗™

Acquisitions manager: Audrey Kaufman; project manager: Joyce Sherman; book and cover design: Matt Avery.

Health Administration Press
A division of the Foundation of the
    American College of Healthcare Executives
One North Franklin Street
Suite 1700
Chicago, IL 60606
(312) 424-2800

Contents

This book is dedicated to a personal hero, Peter Drucker, whose ideas, vision, and brutal candor inspired my career in health management.

Foreword

John P. Glaser, Ph.D., chief information officer,
Partners HealthCare System

FOR 15 YEARS I have had the privilege of being chief information officer for two exceptional organizations: the Brigham and Women's Hospital and Partners HealthCare System. I have also had the honor of serving in several national healthcare information technology (IT) organizations and associations. These experiences have left me with three fundamental observations.

First, without question, much of healthcare delivery does not work very well. Work done by researchers at Partners bears this out. Second, the thoughtful application of IT can undoubtedly lead to significant improvements in healthcare delivery. Third, adoption of IT by providers is low. As few as 5 percent of hospitals have implemented inpatient provider order entry at scale. An estimated 17 percent of primary care providers use a computerized medical record.

Although it might be difficult to argue that healthcare needs to spend as much on IT as the financial services, it would not be difficult to argue that, in aggregate, the investment in IT in healthcare should increase significantly. Such an increase would lead to higher quality, more efficient, and safer healthcare.

Why has this investment not occurred in healthcare organizations? What factors and forces can cause it to occur? Effective application of IT occurs when two major factors are addressed:

1. We must be able to convincingly answer the question posed by solo practitioners, hospitals, and integrated delivery systems, "What's in it for me?" Providers must believe that they need to pursue the implementation of IT.
2. The organization must possess the broad array of assets—for example, leadership, talented teams, and adequate technology—needed to effectively implement these systems.

Clear and compelling evidence exists of a return on the IT investment. This return need not always be increased revenue or reduced costs. It can be in the form of improved service or increased quality of care. However, the return must be seen as important to the organization, and data must be available from organizations "like us" indicating that the return can be achieved.

Regulations and laws require the implementation of some IT applications or related practices. The privacy and transaction code set provisions of HIPAA are examples.

The organization must possess a clear and compelling vision of itself that is enabled by IT. This vision must energize a wide range of leadership, endure over the course of years, and be of sufficient clarity to guide a range of decisions.

Once organizations decide to pursue IT, they must possess, acquire, or develop the assets needed to effectively implement these applications. Asset development falls squarely on the shoulders of the organization's administrative and medical staff leadership and its board.

The first asset is leadership that is smart, honest, seasoned, and committed and that values the healthy exchange of ideas. These leaders want to engage in the IT conversation and, once committed to a course, have the strength to thoughtfully stay that course. They ask hard questions and are pragmatic; they are superb practitioners of the art of the possible.

The second asset is the ability to effect change, at times dramatic change, in work processes, culture, and organizational competencies. This ability requires developing and communicating a vision, political skill in mobilizing stakeholders, stamina, and the willingness to learn. It also means the organizations take steps to mitigate the many factors that often impede their ability to effect change, such as fuzzy goals, poor management of implementations, and failure to put someone in charge.

The third asset is prowess in a small number of critical areas of information systems implementation. Implementation planning needs to be thorough, responsive, and careful. Superb support is the factor that causes an application to "stick," to become an integral part of the fabric of practice. Support includes training, responsive enhancements, ongoing communication and discussion of status and problems, and evolution of work and clinical policies and procedures. Workflow must be thoroughly understood; at times the workflow must be reengineered, and at times the application must be reengineered.

Solid and effective relationships must be established between information systems professionals and users. This relationship is one of realism about the systems and the changes they will bring and one in which there are shared goals and a mutual interest in learning from each other.

The final asset is good IT infrastructure and applications. Clinical information systems must have a technical foundation that is reliable, high performance, secure, supportable, and adaptable. Few things cripple a clinical information system as quickly as a slow or unreliable infrastructure. The applications must also be well designed and managed. Limited ability to enhance applications or augment them with new technologies can result in a poor fit between an application and the clinical workflow and in a failure of the application to adapt as organizations and patient care evolve. Poorly designed applications may not weaken as rapidly as an infrastructure that crashes routinely, but they do weaken.

Information technology is an extraordinarily potent contributor to our collective efforts to improve the delivery of healthcare. Achieving this potential falls largely on the shoulders of the leadership of organizations that make decisions to invest and then pursue the implementation of IT. However, this leadership cannot do this alone. All segments of the healthcare industry must work together and contribute for this vision to occur. Failing to aggressively pursue IT means that, in effect, we accept the state of healthcare as it is today. No one would declare the current system to be satisfactory.

Jeff Goldsmith's book makes a superb contribution to the national undertaking of intelligently applying IT to improve the healthcare delivery system. Jeff has an exquisite, incisive, wide-ranging, and thoughtful mind. He has the remarkable ability to clearly and insightfully write about exceptionally complex topics. This book demonstrates this talent.

Jeff paints a vivid and compelling vision of an IT-enabled healthcare system. He describes emerging information technologies and challenges to our ability to deliver superb healthcare. Jeff highlights the convergence of these technologies and these challenges and sets the stage for a new era of healthcare.

This book will serve its readers well as they lead their organizations into this new era.

Preface

THIS BOOK EMERGED from two parallel learning experiences in the late 1990s: attempting to forecast the impact of the Internet on the health system and learning about healthcare informatics as a new board member of a successful information technology (IT) firm. As a veteran of healthcare strategy and management, I had avoided IT because it was such a quagmire, a field that had struggled, seemingly, for decades to create any measurable value for caregivers or patients. But learning about IT seemed an unavoidable task for anyone seeking to understand and anticipate healthcare's future. What I learned both encouraged and excited me, and you will find the reasons for that excitement in the pages that follow.

The Internet "bubble" created a tremendous stir in equity markets, the media, and society in general before bursting ignominiously in 2000 and taking more than a trillion dollars of investors' capital with it. In healthcare, an immense economic sector that moves very slowly, the Internet was like an unidentified flying object that flew in one window and out the other without even denting the walls, leaving observers wondering what all the fuss was about.

It seemed to me, a relative newcomer to healthcare IT, that the Internet was going to have a significant impact in healthcare, particularly for consumers and health plans, but that it would also take the better part of a generation for healthcare institutions and professionals to adopt and use all the tools affordable connectivity brought them. This seems today like a reasonable forecast.

As I surveyed the technology, however, I became convinced that several innovations would have a more powerful impact on reshaping healthcare institutions and the processes of medicine themselves than the Internet. Moreover, these innovations—computer-assisted molecular and cellular diagnosis, computerized clinical decision support and artificial intelligence, telemedicine (enabling diagnosis of and intervention in illness from a distance), wireless and mobile computing applications, as well as affordable connectivity through the broadband Internet—were converging in a single complex new tool, the so-called "electronic medical record."

This tool is misnamed. As it develops in the next decade, it will not be a historic record of what was done to patients (enabling providers to bill for their services) so much as a navigational tool for physicians and the care team to help them guide patients and their families to a healthier place.

Because healthcare is such a complex and fragmented field, the rapidity with which IT is advancing in a given corner is not apparent to denizens of the other corners. To forecast where these technologies are headed and how they will affect the major actors in health system—hospitals, physicians, consumers, and health plans—seemed like a worthy subject for a book.

The purpose of this book is to provide a panoramic view of IT innovation in healthcare, and more audaciously, a vision of how our health system will look and feel when we have learned how to use all these powerful new tools.

After framing the problems IT can solve in healthcare, the book looks at the technologies themselves and the relationships among them. It then explores how emerging information technologies will affect hospitals, physicians, consumers, and health plans and how their relationships will change as they take up and use these new tools. All these actors crave a more satisfying role in the healthcare process and yet will not, in some unqualified way, embrace important changes that they do not understand or do not believe will help them.

The book also examines the growing absence of fit between our healthcare payment framework and other policies and the emerging capacity to organize healthcare digitally. It discusses what policymakers need to do to speed the transformation in the healthcare system and the leadership challenge involved in bringing about that transformation.

This book is not a utopian exercise. The technologies discussed herein are real, and their potential for helping create a more responsive, safer, and more effective health system is enormous. However, technology sometimes masquerades as an end in itself. Disciplining technology and those who create it to meet our needs is the ultimate task of leadership.

Health services are the most complex commodity our economy produces. Creating modern digital tools to automate major portions of this process may be the most daunting challenge the IT industry has ever faced.

But there is another, more important challenge than the technical one. To achieve the transformation in healthcare that society deserves will require enlightened leadership—in the health professions and healthcare management and from government policymakers. It will also require a willingness on the part of healthcare practitioners and managers to understand and master the technologies themselves—to adapt them, play with them, and collaborate with those who create them—to make them easier to adopt and use.

Leadership is the essential ingredient needed to transform the health system. This book seeks to inspire a new generation of healthcare professionals and managers to understand, master, and deploy these powerful new tools. A better, safer, more effective health system awaits us. It will not happen by itself.

Jeff Goldsmith
May 2003

Acknowledgments

MANY PEOPLE ASSISTED in making this book possible. Neal Patterson, chairman and founder of Cerner Corporation, a pioneering healthcare informatics firm, opened the door by inviting me to serve on Cerner's board of directors. Many Cerner associates, notably Glenn Tobin, Jeff Townsend, and David McCallie, provided valuable insights into systems architecture and the challenges of implementing complex IT solutions. Gartner, the IT consulting and industry research firm, provided numerous opportunities to learn by inviting me to participate in their exceptional healthcare industry forums. Gartner executives and analysts Jim Adams, Dave Garets (now of HealthLink), Janice Young, Thomas Handler, Wes Rishel, and Ken Kleinberg all contributed knowledge and ideas for this book.

Peter Kongstvedt of Cap Gemini Ernst & Young proved a valuable resource on HIPAA and its pivotal role in encouraging IT renovation in healthcare, as well as on health plans' adoption of new technologies. Christine Malcolm, formerly of Computer Sciences Corporation, now of Rush-Presbyterian–St. Luke's Medical Center in Chicago, also provided advice and insights into the challenges of implementing new IT solutions in healthcare payment. David Brailer, CEO of CareScience, helped me understand the challenges of implementing evidence-based medicine using sophisticated IT tools.

On the hospital side, John Glaser, chief information officer at Partners HealthCare in Boston; David Blumenthal, director at the Institute for Health Policy and Physician at The Massachusetts General Hospital/Partners HealthCare System; and Michael Koetting, vice president of planning at the University of Chicago Hospitals, were kind enough to read the manuscript and offer valuable advice on how to make it clearer, sharper, and more relevant.

By happy coincidence, the University of Virginia is a hotbed of medical informatics activity and thought. Several Charlottesville colleagues helped early in the process to shape the book's premise and focus on physicians. They included Don Detmer, former vice chancellor of health affairs at the University of Virginia and now Dennis Gillings Professor of Health Management at Cambridge University in England; William Detmer, CEO of Unbound Medicine, William Knaus, chair of the University of Virginia's Department of Health Evaluation Sciences; and Marshall Ruffin, CEO of Ruffin Informatics, Inc. Robin Felder, professor of pathology and director of the University of Virginia's Medical Automation Research Center, helped me understand the rapid advances in remote sensing technology and their future role in preventive health.

On the scientific front, a fellow Cerner board member, William Neaves, president of the Stowers Institute; Paul Berg, professor emeritus of Stanford University; and George Poste, former chief scientific officer of Smith Kline Beecham, helped shed light on advances in genetic diagnosis. Steven Burrill of Burrill and Company, a biotechnology investment bank, has produced superb analyses of the role of information technology in advancing genetic diagnosis and therapy.

Finally, Anita Gupta ably assisted in the research on this book and the editing and preparation of this manuscript. Laurel Olson also assisted with the initial research and editing. Audrey Kaufman and Joyce Sherman of Health Administration Press provided valuable editorial comments and guidance.

Introduction:
Healthcare Transformed

DAVID SANDY'S STORY

October 28, 2013

When David Sandy woke up on a beautiful fall Monday morning at 6 a.m., his computer was already wide awake. On his home page, in a special medical alert window, he found a reminder message from his physician, Dr. Deborah Kumar, telling him that he needed to send her some bloodwork. David, a 46-year-old computer software engineer, was in radiantly good health and had not seen his physician in 11 months. The reminder was part of a subscription agreement he had negotiated with her last year and was sent him automatically by Dr. Kumar's office computer system.

Part of this agreement was a schedule of periodic monitoring of his health based on his genetic risk profile of potential health risks, including periodic blood tests. David did not need to leave his chair to have his blood analyzed; he simply placed his forefinger on a special touchpad attached to his office computer. A tiny laser beam in the touchpad scanned the blood particles passing through a capillary in his finger and digitally scanned his blood.

The stream of digital information from David's finger was instantly transmitted to the clinical laboratory in Dr. Kumar's hospital, Springfield Memorial, through David's broadband Internet connection. The identification and routing of his bloodwork was preset by the hospital's computer system. This and all of David's other medical information was protected by an elaborate security system designed to shield both the sample and test results from scrutiny by anyone except David and his doctors.

In the hospital's laboratory, a sophisticated image recognition software program automatically read the image of David's blood, counting and categorizing the different blood cells and comparing them to a visual template of normal blood. By 7:30 a.m., the laboratory messaged Dr. Kumar on her cell phone/PDA that it had found a concentration of malformed white blood cells in David's blood and attached a still video clip showing her a high-resolution image. David appeared to have very early stage leukemia. Dr. Kumar received her alert while she was eating breakfast at home and called David to ask if she could drop by to talk with him on her way to the office.

Her PDA also displayed the clinical guideline she and her colleagues at the hospital had agreed to follow, which urged commencing chemopreventive therapy upon laboratory verification of disease and consulting a hematologist on the next steps. Her PDA also indicated, based on a review of her patient records, that she had not seen a leukemic patient in $2\frac{1}{2}$ years, and it listed a series of articles and bulletins on new therapeutic options that would be available to her on her office and home computer "Your Practice Today" homepage in the "You Should Know" section. These articles would bring her up to date on new research findings and innovative therapeutic alternatives for the disease.

When Dr. Kumar arrived at David's house, he took her into his study and listened while Dr. Kumar explained what the lab had found and what it meant. She beamed a copy of the video clip of his blood to David's computer by an infrared signal from her PDA, and he could clearly see the abnormal white cells on his computer monitor.

David was alarmed, although he knew that great strides had been made recently in leukemia treatment and that he was in good hands. Dr. Kumar reassured David that the count of abnormal white cells was still quite low, and based on what she knew, if laboratory analysis confirmed the tentative diagnosis, chemoprevention would probably be the most effective first response. Dr. Kumar asked David if she could draw a sample of David's blood to bring to the hospital laboratory to confirm or rule out the diagnosis.

David asked numerous questions about leukemia, and Dr. Kumar answered them the best she could. She told him that later that morning, he would learn a lot more by reading the attachments to her e-mail about their visit. Those attachments included a primer on the illness, a list of readings on its origins and treatment options, hypertext links to web sites on leukemia, as well as addresses of discussion groups for patients and families undergoing treatment for his disease. She also requested David's permission to discuss his case with Dr. Richard Salerno, Springfield's foremost hematologist and medical oncologist.

With David still in the room, Dr. Kumar located the consultant screen on her PDA, selected Dr. Salerno's name from the consulting list, and with a touch of her stylus directed the hospital's medical record system to transmit an abstract of David's record and a summary of the new laboratory results to Dr. Salerno's PDA, with a voice request for his review of the record and the results of the laboratory analysis.

While driving to her office, Dr. Kumar received a call from Dr. Salerno. He recommended that Dr. Kumar direct the Springfield Memorial Hospital clinical laboratory to copy him on David's blood analysis. If the analysis confirmed the presence of leukemia, Dr. Salerno requested that Dr. Kumar arrange a three-way face-to-face meeting to discuss the treatment options and secure David's permission to begin chemoprevention, the first step in the treatment process.

Meanwhile, Springfield Memorial's clinical laboratory analyzed David's blood sample that morning with flow cytometry, a sophisticated, computer-guided cell-sorting tool; confirmed the diagnosis of leukemia; extracted a sample of leukemic cells from his blood; and isolated a genetic "fingerprint" of David's leukemia to facilitate a possible second defense against the disease.

When Dr. Salerno was notified by computer alert of the confirmation, he scheduled a meeting with David and Dr. Kumar for Tuesday morning in his office. At that meeting, Dr. Salerno explained his view of the case and reviewed the consensus care pathway for David's condition on his office computer. He then summarized his recommendations to David and Dr. Kumar and promised to e-mail David a series of web site links and a record summary to obtain a second opinion electronically from an array of international cancer centers if he wished to do so. David elected to commence chemopreventive therapy.

Shortly after the meeting, Dr. Salerno directed the hospital's pharmacy by computer to prepare a chemopreventive infusion for David based on an analog of retinoic acid (a cousin of vitamin A). If it worked, this infusion would redirect the growth pathway of David's leukemic cells, robbing them of their immortality. The infusion was delivered to David's house by a home infusion therapy team from the hospital the following morning (Wednesday). From the time of diagnosis to commencing therapy, less than 48 hours had elapsed. Every day for the next three weeks, David would receive home infusion therapy, markedly strengthening David's natural immune response to the disease.

Meanwhile, David found a sympathetic reception in the online support group for leukemia patients and spent several hours a day online reading, searching, and asking and answering questions about his situation from new friends he found online. He also had several visits from his mother and sister, whom he had notified immediately of his problem.

Every afternoon, David sent another "movie" of his blood to the Springfield Memorial lab to find out how his leukemia was responding. Meanwhile, the hospital's clinical laboratory was able to compare the genetic fingerprint of David's leukemia via broadband Internet connection with the National Cancer Institute's computer library of known leukemia strains.

Sadly, David's leukemia was a rare and extremely aggressive strain, which was known to resist chemoprevention. This finding triggered an alert to Drs. Salerno and Kumar, with a recommendation that more aggressive therapy for David's cancer begin immediately.

David received an e-mail alert from Dr. Kumar telling him to expect a call from Dr. Salerno requesting that David visit him on Thursday. When David and Dr. Salerno met with Dr. Kumar, Dr. Salerno told him about the problem and indicated that he wanted to request the pharmacogenomics laboratory at Memorial Sloan Kettering Cancer Center in New York to assist in evaluating his condition and in creating a customized therapy to fight his unique cancer.

With David's and Dr. Kumar's concurrence, the pertinent parts of David's medical record, the laboratory record of the genotype of David's cancer, and Dr. Salerno's request for consultation were sent electronically to Sloan Kettering's pharmacogenomics laboratory. A sample of David's blood was sent to New York by overnight courier, arriving a little more than four days after David's initial blood "movie" was taken. The laboratory at Sloan Kettering isolated one of David's leukemic cells through flow cytometry, amplified its DNA, and screened the specific genetic sequences in David's cell that were known to control gene expression.

From this genetic sequence, Sloan Kettering's pharmacogenomics laboratory used a sophisticated computer program and RNA sequencer to fabricate a template of short-strand interfering RNA (RNAi) that could prevent a select few of David's leukemic genes from expressing, thus blocking the replication of David's leukemia. The model RNAi sequence was spliced into *e coli* bacteria cells in Sloan Kettering's laboratory. These cells were then cultured, and RNAi was extracted from them in therapeutic amounts.

The pharmacogenomics laboratory also used a clinical microarray, a miniature clinical laboratory on a computer chip, to inventory the receptors on the surface of David's leukemic cells. Based on the pattern of receptors and a library of similar receptors known to control cancer cell replication, the laboratory created a computer model of the antibody that would most effectively block replication in David's leukemic cells, and sent the data on this protein to the Sloan Kettering antibody fabrication facility.

This antibody was blended with the RNAi into a cocktail of therapeutic compounds, and the resulting IV mixture was sent overnight in a refrigerated container directly to David's house to be added to the infusion therapy regimen prescribed by David's doctors. It arrived three weeks after David's initial diagnosis. On David's computer, he found a message from Sloan Kettering thanking him for seeking their help, as well as a detailed work flow sheet showing what had been done to his blood, and some articles on the technologies they used to craft a personalized response to his leukemia.

The message also contained a short video clip showing what the intended effect of the new therapy was to be. A summary of the Pharmcogenomics Laboratory recommendations and schematic diagrams showing the substances it created were e-mailed to Drs. Salerno and Kumar, along with a set of treatment milestones and tolerances which would guide the administration of David's therapy.

Every day, Springfield's clinical laboratory electronically updated Drs. Kumar and Salerno on David's progress, based on his daily blood movie. Every five days, a home health aide drew a sample of David's blood for the hospital's lab to analyze. Happily, after three weeks of the enhanced therapy, the blood work indicated that David's blood was completely clear of leukemia. Recommended surveillance was cut back to once a week. His physicians sent him a basket of oranges and a note wishing him luck with his work.

David never spent a day in the hospital, and had one home and two office visits with his physicians during the course of treatment, which consisted in its entirety of six weeks' worth of home infusion therapy. The bill for all of these services was created, evaluated, and paid electronically, with David's nominal portion of the cost billed to his Visa card, per agreement with his health plan. He never saw a paper bill, though he could view the billing process in real time on his health plan's web site.

This may seem a fantastic and unreal story, but the technologies to make this story realizable already exist or are under development today. The American health system is on the brink of a fundamental transformation made possible by information technology. That transformation will be costly and complex to achieve, but when it has been accomplished, our relationship to the health system and our ability to manage our own health will be dramatically improved.

Healthcare's clinicians are virtually drowning in information, not only about the illnesses they trained to fight, but also about the process of caring for patients. Much of that information is in paper form, inaccessible or unusable when they need it. This is about to change. The health system, and the information imprisoned in it, is becoming digital. When that digital transformation is complete, vital information about our health and our specific treatment options will be freed from books, paper medical records, and practitioner memories and become moveable to the point of care or to the patient, literally at the speed of light.

The technologies will not, by themselves, change the health system. The American health system is dauntingly complex and bureaucratic. Perhaps more than any other type of innovation, information technology (IT) disturbs existing behavior patterns, workflows, power relationships, and old habits. Digital information is an anarchic force, and its effects are difficult to predict. Moreover, many of these tools are complex, difficult to install, and difficult to learn to use. Information technology is also expensive, and not all healthcare enterprises have the resources to experiment with or invest aggressively in IT.

However, a health system flexible and powerful enough to accommodate individual needs, and to collaborate with us in improving health, is within realization. A safer health system that makes thoughtful, efficient use of the flood of new knowledge, and that is responsive not only to the needs of consumers, but to its workers' values, aspirations, and intellectual curiosity is on the near horizon. This book will help all who work in and use the American health system to understand how to make this achievable future—a more responsive, safer, and more intelligent health system—happen.

CHAPTER 1

The Information Quagmire

IF YOU BELIEVE, with Peter Drucker, that the core product of a modern society is knowledge, the American health system is the world's largest, most complex, and most dynamic knowledge enterprise.[1] It specializes in knowledge of the most profound and intimate sort—how long and how well people will live, what ails them, and how they can influence their well-being using medical science's increasingly powerful toolbox.

In fact, this knowledge enterprise, the American health system, is the size of a large industrial nation. At more than $1.3 trillion, it was larger in 2000 than the gross domestic product (GDP) of France or China and nearly four times the size of all the African economies combined (Figure 1.1). Yet from the standpoint of the use of modern information technology (IT), the American health system is still very much a third world country. Despite the investment of tens of billions of dollars in information systems, the more than 12 million caregivers and support personnel in the most technologically advanced health system in the world are buried in a blizzard of paper and flurries of unreturned telephone calls.

I began my work in healthcare in late 1975 at the University of Chicago's Medical Center, a 700-bed urban teaching hospital. My most vivid memory of the orientation tour was visiting the hospital's medical records room. It was an enormous room in the basement, stacked floor to ceiling with dusty telephone book–sized paper medical records.

Dozens of workers protected from the dust by white coats moved piles of these bulging records around the hospital in shopping carts. With so much paper and such haphazard filing, tracking charts inside the two-million-square-foot University of Chicago medical complex was a massive and frustrating logistical challenge. Failure to locate and deliver charts to the clinics and inpatient units delayed or hampered the care process, resulting in increased cost and frustration for patients, nurses, and physicians alike.

That medical records room reminded me of nothing so much as the municipal library in the capital of an underdeveloped country— a record-keeping system more appropriate to Dickens' London than a modern enterprise. Although the University of Chicago hospital system has subsequently invested millions of dollars in electronic records systems, as well as more capacious plastic shopping carts, the records room, jammed with medicine's biblical stone tablets, is still there today in 2003. Virtually every contemporary American hospital has such a room.

Despite breathtaking advances in other sectors of the American economy in applying digital information and communications technologies, medical decision making at the dawn of the twenty-first century remains unhappily yoked to paper, the telephone, and practitioners' memories. Paper medical records, often unreadable paper prescriptions, paper orders, paper lab reports, paper telephone message slips, fax paper health insurance verifications, paper bills of questionable accuracy: these are the artifacts of an early 1970s information environment.

Not that hospitals and other clinical enterprises lack computers.

Figure 1.1: Gross Domestic Products, 2000

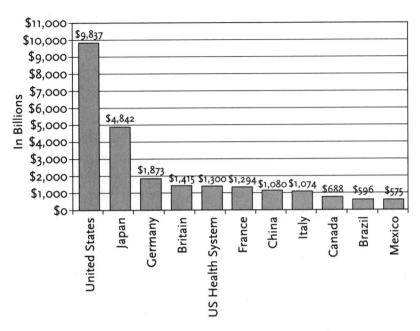

Source: *The Economist: Pocket in World Figures* (2003), New York: John Wiley and Sons; Health Care Financing Administration, Office of the Actuary (2001).

On the contrary, hospitals are filled with them. Sheldon Doren-fest estimates that, once the tally is in, the health IT market will have continued to rise and IT expenditures will be $23.5 billion in 2003.[2] Almost every desk has a computer, but this pervasive presence has not resulted in practical or efficient record keeping and use. A typical large American hospital may have as many as three dozen separate computer systems, ranging in age from near-Technicolor-quality youth to green-screened senility. The software used in these systems is written in different code, operates on different hardware platforms, and may be maintained (often inadequately) by a dozen or more different vendors whose systems do not, to use IT jargon for compatibility, "interoperate." The typical health enterprise is an informational "Tower of Babel."

Although patients may imagine themselves to be a single, unitary person, many large medical enterprises see those individuals as up to a dozen different persons, depending on which and how many parts of the enterprise they encounter. That is, a patient may be a different person in the emergency room than he or she is in the clinical laboratory, in the surgical suite, and yet again in the doctor's office just a day earlier. Each of these different sites of care within the same organization maintains a different medical record of its encounters with same patient. These separate systems were primarily built to bill for each department's services, not to guide patient care.

There is also a nearly impermeable barrier between the hospital's records and those of the physicians who direct the care. In the typical community hospital, it is impossible for the doctor or any other care worker to access the doctor's office records from any site other than that doctor's office because more than 80 percent of those office records are still in paper form. Furthermore, most doctors in private medical practice have been unwilling to support shared digital record-keeping systems with their hospitals because of a profound lack of trust and poor communication with hospital management.

Even where it is possible to link all of these fragments of a patient's history and medical situation electronically, a considerable feat of software engineering is required to move this information around quickly enough that it can actually be used by the physician in making important care decisions. When information reaches a digital dead end, it is printed out and piled up in various in-boxes or paper filing systems. Thus, vital information remains locked up in paper, or in people's short-term memories, and cannot flow through wire or fiber or the air to where it is needed to make timely and accurate medical decisions.

As long as the source documents detailing patient care remain in paper form, the only way to determine whether particular clinical decisions contributed to a positive health outcome is to hire squads of graduate students or nurses to cull the records by hand months later and tabulate the results. The fact that we know so little about what actually works in medical treatment can be attributed in large part to the prison of paper we have constructed around the care process.

THE FLOOD OF NEW MEDICAL KNOWLEDGE

As if these logistical challenges were not enough to hinder the care decision process, new knowledge and new technologies based on that knowledge are flooding the health system. Public research investments through the National Institutes of Health and private equity investment, including research and development expenditures by the nation's pharmaceutical and biotechnology firms, are creating new medical knowledge at a stunning pace.

In 2001, nearly $51 billion was invested in creating new knowledge in medicine just in the United States.[3] This amount compares favorably to the GDP of a medium-sized Latin American country and results in the generation of almost 60,000 new citations *monthly* in the National Library of Medicine's MEDLINE research service.[4] Organizing and disseminating this flood of new knowledge to a "community" of nearly 700,000 active physicians is a huge logistical and "knowledge management" challenge.

The logistics of medical practice itself have become so dauntingly complex that physicians barely have time for their families, let alone time to keep pace with the exciting advances in their own fields. A monthly continuing medical education session at the hospital or local medical society and periodic visits from pharmaceutical salespeople are the principal conduits of new knowledge to most practicing physicians.

A visit to a physician's personal office typically reveals piles of unread medical journals, pink telephone message slips, and scattered samples of new drugs from the last pharmaceutical sales representative to visit the office. The computer in the office is probably turned off, is likely at least three years old, and is surely not configured to reach or retain data about current medical practice. Physicians know they are not keeping up, and this both frustrates and frightens them.

Professional training and culture in medicine conditioned physicians to rely principally on direct peer contact and what they can carry around in their memories to support their advice to patients. The channels by which new information reaches physicians in practice are dangerously narrow and lack the bandwidth and intelligence to organize and transmit the flood of new medical knowledge in a way that it can be absorbed and used in practice. Although major journals have digitized their articles and made them available online, medical knowledge is still largely paper driven. Unless physicians have a good relationship with a medical librarian or, as do a lucky few senior physicians in teaching hospitals, have residents and fellows to research issues for them, the large number of important questions about a patient's health that occur to a physician during a typical practice day never get answered.

FAILING THE CRUCIAL TEST—
DELIVERING SAFE AND SATISFACTORY CARE

The outdated record-keeping systems and lack of time to stay current with the flood of information would be excusable if the health system was safe and actually worked to meet consumer needs. However, the reality is that the lack of timely and accurate information at the point of care is a major contributor to patient deaths and injuries, as well as resulting in a waste of time and money.

In a landmark study published in 2000 entitled *To Err is Human*, the Institute of Medicine (IOM) of the National Academy of Science reported that as many as 98,000 patients die annually in the nation's hospitals as a result of medical errors.[5] The IOM report cites poor coordination of care and lack of modern information systems as major contributors to exposing patients to risk. (It does not, as some publishers in the popular press may be tempted to do, advocate seeking out "bad" doctors and nurses for blame.)

In addition to the quality issue, although most Americans continue to express confidence in their physicians and hospitals, consumer satisfaction with the overall health system is declining. As a vehicle for applying medical knowledge to solving problems, the healthcare system has become increasingly cumbersome, user-unfriendly, and expensive.

When the Internet opened up new channels for consumers to access medical knowledge directly, it was rapidly flooded with users. According to a recent Harris poll, roughly 110 million Americans used the Internet to seek health information in 2002.[6] This explosion of Internet use was an expression of consumer frustration with the current system of transmitting medical knowledge.

WHY HAVE HEALTH SERVICES RESISTED MODERN IT?

Why do health services lag 20 years or more behind other industries in using IT to improve safety, efficiency, and customer service? There are many reasons. Healthcare is the most complex product our economy produces. Even small healthcare institutions are complex, barely manageable places. According to Peter Drucker (see Note 1), large healthcare institutions, like urban academic health centers, may be the most complex organizations in human history.

Not only do the medical problems presented at the point of service vary tremendously, but no inventory exists; health services are, for the most part, custom manufactured for individual patients on a "just in time" basis. For most healthcare, there is no template on which physicians can rely to make decisions about health. This is because professional consensus on what best practice is or ought to be is only now emerging.

Perhaps most significantly, more complex, highly trained health professionals collide at the point of care than in any other business in our economy. Each profession has its own unique view of the patient's needs, its own language for describing those needs, and an intensely territorial view of its involvement in care. Collaboration among professionals is vital to effective care, yet professions compete for resources and control over patients. Systemic innovations like IT that foster or even demand collaboration or that systematize treatment decisions face difficult hurdles to adoption.

CHANGE IS IN THE AIR

Information technology in medicine is nearing the end of a lengthy and troubled adolescence. It is on the verge of revolutionizing medical practice, dramatically improving communication among physicians and between physicians and patients. Spurred not only by continued advances in hardware, but also by breakthroughs in software and network architecture, IT has matured to the point where it will make a major difference for consumers as well as physicians and other caregivers.

Whereas hospitals and major insurers have been connected electronically for years through dedicated, high-bandwidth telephone conduits called T1 lines, the advent of the Internet has recently brought affordable broadband connect ivity to doctors and patients. The Internet has not only brought new options for physicians and patients to connect with one another, it has made possible connectivity to and networking with thousands of colleagues and tens of thousands of patients worldwide. Some specific technologies are discussed below.

ASP

Using a technology called application service provision (ASP), complex software can now be delivered through the Internet for practitioners and institutions that cannot afford multimillion-dollar systems installations. Complex software can now be maintained efficiently at a single site on remote servers, which hospital and physician users can reach by way of a web browser and high-speed

Internet connections. Clinical and financial information can be sent rapidly to remote locations and returned to the institutions or caregivers that need it to make care decisions.

Although ASP has gotten off to a slow start, this technology will eventually remove the financial and complexity barriers to obtaining sophisticated computer support for clinical care wherever it is needed. This means that eventually, small-scale clinical operations, like physicians' offices, rural health clinics, community health centers, and small hospitals, will have access to the same powerful applications as wealthy institutions with large IT staffs.

XML

Improvements in an obscure but vital software utility called mark-up language will make searching the Internet for and finding disease-specific or patient-specific information easier. A computer language called XML (or *extensible mark-up language*) creates "smart" tags for information contained in web sites, which facilitate the location of medical information by search engines, medical librarians, professionals, and consumers. XML enables the Internet user to locate and retrieve information based on what it means, rather than how it is supposed to look on a web page. It markedly reduces the time and cost of finding answers to medical questions on the Internet and may be more important to medicine than any other knowledge domain. XML also has the ability to convert the nearly 100 million pages of web-based medical information from a vast, opaque magazine rack to a searchable database of medical knowledge.

Computer-assisted Diagnosis

Computer-assisted diagnosis will penetrate into the nucleus of human cells, providing an extraordinarily detailed and highly personal map of a patient's potential health risks, including the risks of various forms of therapy. This in turn will enable the custom fabrication of therapies to control unique risks for disease and adverse reactions to treatment and eventually extinguish diseases before they flower into illness or threaten our lives. Genetic information will play a part in computer-assisted diagnosis, enabling physicians to reduce adverse drug reactions, adjust dosages to an optimal therapeutic result, and avoid wasting drugs on patients who are unlikely to respond to them. Genetic information will become an essential part of our health records and help provide a basis for a new, exquisitely personal, and proactive form of medicine.

Powerful computing engines have dramatically enhanced mature diagnostic imaging technologies like magnetic resonance imaging and computed tomography. These technologies can today create live, three-dimensional images of internal organs that provide not only vivid anatomical detail, but also indicate whether the organs are functioning properly. These imaging technologies will be powerful enough to detect threatening molecular and genetic changes in our cells as they are occurring. Thanks to growing broadband Internet capacity and internal communications networks (or intranets), digital images and their interpretations can be moved, literally at light speed, to the desktops of clinicians anywhere in the world without being translated into film or paper.

AI

Perhaps the most exciting advances are those in artificial intelligence (AI) and expert systems in medicine. Almost 30 years of frustrating progress in medical informatics are yielding promising new "intelligent" clinical applications that will save both lives and dollars. Computer systems that can communicate with clinicians, patients, and patients' families and respond intelligently to the health risks they confront are within realization.

Intelligent clinical information systems will be continuously aware of a patient's condition and will alert the care team to problems as they arise, as well as recommend courses of action to achieve the best outcome. Clinical information systems will no longer passively record what physicians do. Rather, they will actively shape the care process, providing a "navigational system" for guiding care and a "flight plan" for improving health. This plan will be transparent, accessible to patients and their families, and customizable, enabling the clinical team and patients to examine the studies, data, and justifications for recommended care.

Dissemination and Care-decision Capabilities

Information technology will enable expert medical knowledge to pervade our societies, transcending the constraints of geography, language, and local infrastructure. IT will eventually eliminate much of the wasteful and inefficient clerical and administrative processes that consume a far larger than justifiable share of the nation's healthcare bill.

Most importantly, however, IT will help improve medical care itself, reducing medical errors and providing crucial and timely help in making better care decisions. Finally, information will enable patients and their families to have more control over their own lives and health. It will provide them secure and reliable personal health records and a "dashboard" on their home computer's web browser that will help them manage their relationship to their doctors, hospitals, pharmacies, and the rest of the health system.

CONCLUSION

Because the healthcare system is so vast and fragmented, it is easy for people operating in one corner of it to be unaware of the impact IT is having on the rest of the system. The technologies you will learn more about in this book—electronic medical records, clinical decision support, genetic diagnosis, medical imaging, telemedicine, digital business systems in health insurance and health systems— are all connected by the Internet to one another. The Internet provides both the connectivity for all these different but reinforcing technologies and the lubricant of information flow throughout the health system. The result will be a powerful, capable, and responsive health system.

Between this potential and today's information quagmire stands a huge societal commitment: an expenditure that could exceed $300 billion in the United States alone over the next ten years. Also looming ahead is a monstrous implementation headache. Healthcare organizations of all types face a large skill gap in adapting these powerful new tools and a steep learning curve for the firms providing the technology. However, healthcare institutions and professions must take on the challenge to implement technology, a task that includes the concepts and processes described in this book. Healthcare will be irrevocably changed as it adopts and uses these technologies.

NOTES

1. Drucker, P. 1993. *Post-Capitalist Society*. New York: Harper and Row.

2. Sheldon I. Dorenfest & Associates. 2002. "Healthcare Information Technology Spending is Gaining Momentum in 2002." [Online information; retrieved 1/3/03.] Chicago: Sheldon I. Dorenfest & Associates. www.dorenfest.com/pressrelease .asp.

3. Pharmaceutical Research and Manufacturers of America. 2002. *2002 Industry Profile*. Washington, DC: PhRMA.

4. National Library of Medicine. 2002. "Fact Sheet MedLine." [Online information; retrieved 12/2/02.] Bethesda, MD: www.nlm.nih.gov/pubs/factsheets/medline .html.

5. Kohn, L. T., J. M. Corrigan, and M. S. Donaldson, eds. 2000. *To Err is Human: Building a Safer Health System*. Washington, DC: National Academy Press.

6. Taylor, H., and R. Leitman, eds. 2002. "Cyberchondriacs Continue to Grow in America." *Harris Interactive* 2 (9): 1–4.

CHAPTER 2

Digital Medicine

HEALTHCARE IS IN the midst of a technological transition, the outcome of which has dramatic implications. In the pre-digital age we are leaving, the vital knowledge about medical history and treatment options would have been found imprisoned in paper and film—in the form of multiple medical records, medical texts, and journals—or locked in the memories of those who have recently provided care. The only way for the care team to use this information was to have physical possession of it, read it, and interpret it in an effort to figure out a treatment plan. Furthermore, for care team members to develop and implement such a plan, two or more members typically needed to be on the telephone at the same time or in the same room to coordinate their efforts.

In the digital age we are entering, vital information and knowledge about conditions, as well as how to treat them, will become as mobile as quicksilver. This information will be able to travel anywhere in the world with broadband connectivity at the speed of light. Every piece of this knowledge about patients and the medical problems confronting them will be converted over the next decade from paper and film to digital files. Moreover, to use that knowledge, the only thing that caregivers will need is access to a computer system connected to patients' records.

Each corner of the health system is seeing its own digital revolution. Yet the big picture—the extent of the revolution—has eluded healthcare providers, because they cannot see how all these technologies will come together to change how the care team behaves and how consumers interact with the health system. This chapter explores this convergence by looking at the different knowledge domains—molecular and cellular, tissues and organ systems, care processes—relevant to treatment. It also discusses the technical aspects of care as they evolve and how they will affect healthcare delivery, including remote medicine, the Internet, and electronic medical records. The chapter continues with an examination of a navigation system for clinical care and the prospects for its use by physicians in a teacher/protector role, and it concludes by addressing technical requirements for the digital revolution to continue.

GENOMICS: THE MOST INTIMATE KNOWLEDGE

More than 50 years ago, James Watson and Henry Crick discovered that DNA is the recipe for all life. It is digital software—the most complex software known in the universe—comprising three billion bits of chemical "code" embedded in the nucleus of each cell in the body. This amazing molecule contains not only the template for every one of the hundreds of thousands of proteins in the body, but also the assembly instructions for turning those proteins into a functioning human being.

Most major illnesses troubling patients today, including heart disease, cancer, Alzheimer's disease, and many forms of mental illness, have genetic roots. As Matt Ridley remarks in his poetic and insightful book, *Genome*, genes are not there to cause disease, but to support normal functioning.[1] Understanding *how* genes enable one's body to function properly is the tough challenge facing human geneticists.

High-performance computing that uses diagnostic microchips, computerized cell-sorting machines, computer-guided DNA sequencers, molecular imaging, powerful computing algorithms, and vast DNA databases is playing the decisive role in unraveling the mystery of DNA's influence on health. Genomics *is* information technology; shut down the computers, and modern cell biology rapidly grinds to a halt.

With the completion of the Human Genome Project in late 2000, western society was inundated with a great deal of hype heralding the seemingly immediate impact that mapping the location of all of a person's genes would have on his or her health. It seemed for a brief, giddy moment that a new wave of genetically based cures for disease would shortly be unleashed. Shortly thereafter, however, reality set in. When asked what stood between the gene map and a comprehensive understanding of human disease, one scientist, Dr. William Neaves of the Stowers Institute of Medical Research, responded, "About one hundred years of hard work."[2]

The most complex diseases do have genetic roots, but those roots may comprise hundreds or even thousands of genes. These genes fluidly and continuously interact with a person's environment, his or her behavior, and each other in a bewilderingly complex manner to create disease risk. Translating information about genetic risk of disease into focused prevention, such as gene therapy, that extinguishes disease risk at the molecular level, remains a daunting scientific and technical challenge.

However, one hundred years will not have to pass before genetic information reshapes healthcare. Indeed, it is happening as you read this book. DNA testing is the most rapidly growing segment of a relatively moribund clinical laboratory (e.g., in vitro diagnostic) business. According to Reuters Business Insight, the DNA testing industry conducted $1 billion worth of business worldwide in 2001 and is growing at 35 percent per year (Figure 2.1).[3]

This growth is spurred not by traditional uses, such as predisposition testing for diseases like sickle cell anemia or Huntington's disease or forensic testing to aid criminal investigations. Rather, it

Figure 2.1: Global Market for Genomic Diagnostics, 2000–05

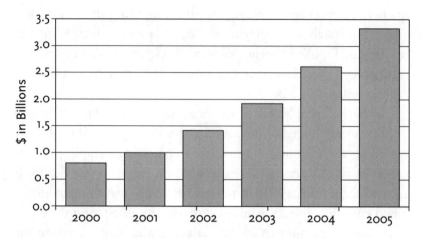

Source: Dooley, J. F. 2002. *The Genomics Outlook to 2005: Transforming Pharmaceutical and Diagnostic Markets.* London: Reuters Business Insight.

is driven by advances in treatment of infectious diseases and cancer, where genetic information is being used to guide treatment decisions with today's therapeutic options.

Genetics and Treatment

Among the first pathogens to be affected by this new technology has been the human immunodeficiency virus (HIV). The key to HIV's virulence is the fact that the virus furiously mutates, seeking to present a camouflage to evade the immune systems' formidable defenses. HIV may evolve through 3,000 generations inside the body during the course of the illness.

DNA testing is being used by HIV treatment teams to find the unique genetic signature of the virus that is present in the bodies of AIDS patients at the moment of testing. This signature is then compared to computer libraries of known strains of the virus that are susceptible or resistant to various drugs in the therapeutic cocktail. By tailoring the elements and dosages in the cocktail to the genetic signature of the virus, far more rapid and efficient clearing of the virus has been achieved.[4,5]

Genetic selectivity is also key to guiding the development and approval of many new and expensive forms of cancer treatment. For example, the federal Food and Drug Administration refused to approve a new drug, Herceptin, targeted to treat breast cancer, until its manufacturer, Genentech, produced a test to determine if breast cancer cells actually displayed the receptor, HER-2, to which Herceptin is targeted. Giving the drug to patients whose cells do not display this receptor means wasting $20,000 on a drug with no clinical effect. Many new drugs will be approved in the next few years conditional upon a genetic test to determine if the therapy is likely to be effective.

Even more exciting than these advances are discoveries that genetic variation may hold the key to predicting the likelihood of an adverse drug reaction (ADR). In 1994 in the United States, an estimated 76,000 hospital patients died from an ADR. If this estimate is accurate, ADRs would constitute the sixth leading cause of death in the United States, after heart disease, cancer, stroke, pulmonary disease, and accidents; this would rank ADRs ahead of pneumonia and diabetes.[6] Researchers in one study found genetic lesions in genes controlling the metabolism (processing by the liver) of 59 percent of major drugs producing adverse reactions—in plainer English, strong circumstantial evidence of a genetic basis of ADRs, which could predict an individual's likelihood of a bad outcome. Assaying these genes, like cytochrome p450, may hold the key to avoiding ADRs in the future.[7]

At the same time, genetic variation may be instrumental in predicting whether a drug has any therapeutic effect on individual patients. For those receiving initial HIV therapy, as many as 60 percent or more of the patients who receive it do not respond.[8] The ability to predict nonresponse may help clinical teams avoid wasting these increasingly precious and expensive resources on patients they do not help.

These uses represent only the beginning of a new era of personalized, genetically customized medicine (Figure 2.2). Within a decade, the genetic signature of a pathogen such as a virus or a cancer cell may form the basis for fabrication of customized therapies, such as vaccines, specifically targeted at that pathogen. Clinical laboratories will use genetic information to identify targets on the cell surface or in the nucleus of the pathogen that can be blocked by antibodies or by agents that retard or prevent dangerous genes from expressing in the first place.[9,10]

Eventually, predisposition testing will evaluate the genetic disease risks buried in genetic makeup and give the clinical team information to correct or override defective genetic information that threatens lives and health. Progress in gene therapy has been hampered, however, by the vigor of the immune response to new genetic material introduced into the body, as well as by an inability to target new genetic information to the right places in the genome. Control over expression of disease-causing pathogens or genes may be a more achievable goal than inserting the "correct" genetic information.[11]

Changing Roles of Clinicians

Just as radiologists morphed from being pure diagnosticians to clinicians who intervene in peripheral vascular disease or in strokes, clinical pathology will acquire a curative dimension in the next decade. This curative role will be the result of molecular information technologies—microarrays and computerized cell sorting, principally—focused on acquiring genetic information about the patient and the pathogen. Pathologists will also find themselves competing in genetic diagnosis with the radiologists as they develop molecular imaging technology.

Figure 2.2: Genetics and Medicine—Phases of Adoption of "Personalized Medicine"

1. Genotyping as basis for therapeutic selection (0–7 years)
   • screening out adverse responders or non-responders
   • setting therapeutic mix based on pathogen genotype
2. Genotyping as basis for customized vaccination/ therapies (8–15 years)
3. Predisposition testing leading to genetic therapy or controlled gene expression (15 years plus)

Source: Burrill, S. 2001. *Biotech 2001: Life Sciences: Genomics, Proteonomics . . . and More.* The Biotechnology Industry 15th Annual Report. San Francisco: Burrill and Company.

Impact on Health Systems

The ability to use genetic information to guide and craft therapy will become a key differentiator of hospitals and health centers within the next decade, much as open-heart surgery was during the 1970s. Personalized medicine based on genetic testing represents the leading edge of a huge new service opportunity for our nation's health system, as well as a powerful tool set for making drug therapy safer and more effective.

ANALYZING OUR CELLS, TISSUES, AND ORGAN SYSTEMS

Modern computer technologies have enabled rapid advances both in clinical laboratory and radiological analysis of disease. Previously, the output of these analyses was paper notes with line drawings, x-ray film, and pathology slides. Today, the analyses are in digital form, and the results can be stored, retrieved, and sent electronically.

Tomorrow, the initial diagnosis process (e.g., Is there a malignant lesion in the breast? Is the cell infected with a virus? If so, what virus?) will be performed by computer software, with physician overreading to confirm the diagnosis. Diagnostic results will flow seamlessly through the so-called "electronic medical record" into structured and timely recommendations to the care team.

Diagnostic Tools

Sir Arthur C. Clarke once said that at some level of sophistication, technology is indistinguishable from magic. Today's digitally assisted diagnostic tools seem little short of magical.

Flow Cytometry

Flow cytometry enables a laboratory technician to count and sort individual cells flowing through a highly pressurized thread of water up to a rate of up to 70,000 cells per second, plucking single cells of interest (each less than one-twentieth of the width of a human hair) out of the stream with magnetic pulses and dropping them into wells in a laboratory tray.

This remarkable specificity is made possible by computerized interpretation of the diffraction patterns of a laser beam passing through the thread and bouncing off individual cells. The scattered light reaches electronic plates positioned around the stream, which record the pattern of light as digital information. The same technology can detect fluorescent markers on cells that indicate the presence of a particular receptor on the cell surface, or even a particular sequence of DNA in the cell's nucleus.

Using a computer-controlled magnetic pulse, the operator can pluck specific cells from the stream for further analysis. Flow cytometry is powerful enough to detect, for example, fetal cells in a sample of the mother's blood and extract them without the need for invasive and sometimes dangerous amniocentesis. It can also count and categorize cancer cells by their shape or the constellation of receptors on their surface.

After DNA analysis, flow cytometry is the second most rapidly growing clinical laboratory modality, at a more than 20 percent compound growth rate annually.[12] Biologists are hopeful that they can learn to coax human stem cells to grow into replacement tissues or even whole organ systems. If this becomes possible, flow cytometry will be the tool hospitals use to find stem cells in the blood. These cells will be cultured and redirected to therapeutic levels for treating diseases like Parkinson's, diabetes, or spinal cord injury. Because they are cultured from an individual's own cells, the recipient will not require a lifetime of immune suppressants to enable them to do their work.

Modifications to MRI and PET

Diagnostic imaging technologies like computed tomography (CT), magnetic resonance imaging (MRI), ultrasound, and positron emissions tomography (PET) have been in use for almost two generations. They are mature, workhorse technologies, made possible by computerized interpretation of various forms of signals after they pass through the body: x-rays in the case of CT, radiofrequency shifts in the case of MRI, sound waves in the case of ultrasound, and radioactive energy from tracers in the case of PET. In all cases, the signals are detected by digital arrays and converted to digital information structured and stored by computers.

These technologies, revolutionary when they were developed, made noninvasive evaluation of tissues and internal organs possible, tilting diagnosis decisively away from exploratory surgery (and tilting power and clinical influence toward radiology). Computed tomography, magnetic resonance (MR), and ultrasound enabled radiologists to locate damaged tissues; now, MR spectroscopy and PET enable radiologists to determine if tissues are actually alive and whether the organs they constitute are functioning properly.

Magnetic resonance spectroscopy and PET can determine if tissues are metabolizing; that is, they can indicate whether tissues are taking up oxygen and burning calories. These images can reveal the extent of damage to the heart or brain from a heart attack or stroke and help determine if a tumor has been destroyed by radiation or chemotherapy. Some vendors claim that through computerized combination of images from PET and high resolution (multislice) CT, the ability to pinpoint the location of a tumor in the body has improved by 60 percent. In addition, the capability of diagnosing the type of lesion has increased by 40 percent. With molecular imaging, these technologies will actually be able to identify real-time cellular changes or gene expression patterns that prefigure disease.[13]

All these imaging modalities are made possible by a computing engine that digitally reconstructs the acquired signals into vivid images. In the 30 years since they were invented, there has been a logarithmic growth in the computing power of a microchip. This growth in computing power was predicted by Gordon Moore, one of the founders of Intel, in 1967. In one of the most extraordinary (self-fulfilling) predictions in the history of technology, Moore said that the power of a microchip would double every 18 months with cost remaining constant (Figure 2.3).[14]

This extraordinary sustained increase in computing power has enabled a dramatic expansion in the speed and accuracy of diagnostic imaging. More powerful computing engines mean more rapid acquisition of images and more options for manipulating and reconstructing these images. Today, these modalities stand on the brink of eliminating the need for invasive procedures, such as colonoscopy and coronary angiography, and are capable of producing remarkable three-dimensional images of functioning internal organs.[15]

Figure 2.3: Moore's Law—Transistors per Microprocessor

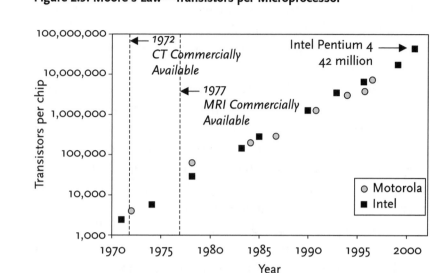

Source: Hackworth, M. 1999. "Now, Software Must Take Over Even if Chips No Longer Follow Moore's Law, Efficiencies Don't Have to End." *San Jose Mercury News,* Oct. 19, 6B. Used with Permission.

Changes in Radiology

Two key changes in radiology—teleradiology and machine interpretation of radiological images—have been made possible by the successful standardization of formats for digital radiological images. Collaboration between the radiology profession and radiology equipment manufacturers produced a data standard called DICOM.[16] Digital images produced by modern radiology equipment anywhere in the world are now constructed and transmitted in this common format.

Inside hospitals and multispecialty clinics, images are sent and stored through computer systems called picture archiving and communication systems (PACS), so they can be viewed and interpreted without having to be converted to film. With the advent of broadband Internet connections, radiological images can not only be transmitted instantaneously inside hospitals or clinics, but they can also be sent virtually anywhere in the world where someone is available to interpret them.

For example, many hospital radiology departments now send digital MR and CT scans through broadband Internet connection to colleagues in India, Australia, or New Zealand, who overread the scans overnight while their colleagues in the United States are sleeping. When U.S. radiologists come into the office the next morning, the interpretations from across the world are available in their communication system to help guide clinical care decisions.[17]

Teleradiology—digital radiology enhanced by broadband Internet connectivity—has removed the geographic constraints on the practice of radiology, setting off unprecedented competition in the field. Teleradiology has created service opportunities for isolated rural hospitals and practitioners who cannot afford full-time subspecialized radiology coverage.

Advances in image recognition software will enable radiology equipment to interpret as well as create radiological images. Recent studies have established that machine-read mammograms detect more lesions and stage them more accurately than do human radiologists.[18] As computerized interpretation becomes more reliable, the software will come installed in new scanners and x-ray modalities or in radiology information systems. Human judgment will be focused on the "tough calls," the machine-identified exceptions that require overreading.

REMOTE MEDICINE: MONITORING AND THERAPY

For at least 20 years, cardiologists in major heart centers have been able to monitor patients with unstable heart rhythms or who are recovering from acute episodes by reading electrocardiograms (EKGs) transmitted through dedicated telephone connections.[19,20,21] The expansion of broadband connectivity and the development of intelligent, programmable monitoring devices taking place now and in the near future will enable cardiologists to monitor ambulatory patients at cardiac risk without either hospitalizing them or connecting them to a telephone.

Remote Monitoring

In Philadelphia recently, a newly formed technology firm, CardioNet, created the first regional wireless network to monitor ambulatory cardiac patients. Working in cooperation with local hospitals and cardiologists, patients are fitted with a three-lead sensor, which communicates with a wearable EKG unit that monitors their heart rhythms. This device is contained in a wireless sending unit the size of a personal digital assistant, which transmits the signals to a base station where human operators are assisted by continuous computer monitoring of their heart rhythms.

If the patient appears to be experiencing cardiac distress, a voice channel will enable the operator to communicate directly with the patient, verify his or her condition orally, and direct him or her to take action. The system automatically alerts the patient's physician to the problem and can even trigger an ambulance call to bring the patient to the hospital if required.[22]

The Sentara Health System in Norfolk, Virginia, has used these same remote monitoring tools to create a four-hospital intensive care unit (ICU) overseen from a remote location by a supervising intensivist. The system is so efficient that a single intensivist assisted by a single nurse is able to monitor 40 ICU patients remotely.[23] (The system will eventually scale up to 200 ICU patients for a single intensivist assisted by a critical care nurse.) The result has been not only a dramatic reduction in cost, but also a 25 percent reduction in mortality rates.[24] Hospitals struggling to cope with high occupancy will discover that these remote monitoring systems can free up beds and nursing staff to cope with the sickest of their patients.

Taking this process to the next step, Medtronic, the technology leader in cardiac pacemakers, has developed an implantable device that monitors, stores, and transmits information about the patient's cardiac rhythm directly to the patient's physician. These devices can be programmed (and reprogrammed remotely) to vary pacing depending on the patient's unique needs and can also administer an electric shock to restart the patient's heart if it moves into atrial fibrillation.[25,26]

Medtronic is developing similar intelligent implantable devices for other organ systems (the brain, the spinal cord, the pancreas, the digestive system, etc.), which can accumulate and process data about bodily processes and communicate that data to monitoring systems wirelessly.[27] Intelligent, interactive implantable devices based on computer technology will provide platforms for clinicians to influence key internal organ systems remotely and in real time.

Progress in miniature sensing technologies is creating a new generation of devices that can be worn or embedded in people's homes to monitor their health noninvasively and automatically alert family or caregivers if problems arise. The "smart shirt," for example, enables monitoring of multiple vital signs (heart rhythms and respiration) and transmittal of aberrant results to family or the care team. These same technologies, when embedded in the home environment, will enable one to determine if an elderly person has fallen, is having trouble breathing, has taken prescribed medications, or is eating.[28] Furthermore, the "smart house" project is wedding sophisticated sensor technologies to computerized monitoring to create a safe environment at home as an alternative to institutionalizing elderly people.[29,30] In all these cases, intelligent monitoring systems are extending the protective reach of the clinical team while eliminating the need to institutionalize patients.

Remote Surgery

Wedding broadband connectivity to sophisticated imaging software is enabling even surgical procedures to be done from remote locations. In November 1999, clinicians in New York City made history by successfully performing a colecystectomy on a patient in Strasbourg, France.[31] The surgeon in New York was able to manipulate a laparoscope inserted into the abdomen of the patient in France via a video feed and robotic connection. These same technologies will enable students to learn via "virtual" surgical procedures using interactive software that reflects to them real world images of internal organs. Telepresence technologies are producing live, three-dimensional images of internal organs, which enable physicians and their students to "tour" the body of a patient virtually.[32]

Although robotic surgery (enabling surgeons to perform extremely fine movements in neurosurgical and cardiac procedures with computer assistance) presently requires surgeons to be in the same room as the patient, technologists working for the Department of Defense have been perfecting the same technologies to enable surgeons in rear areas to operate on injured soldiers in hot zones by way of telepresence.[33]

Voice Recognition

Finally, impressive progress in speech recognition and natural language processing are enabling clinical teams and health plans to interact with patients over the telephone. Voice response technologies are likely to play an important, augmenting role in connecting patients and people at risk to the health system. During the Internet frenzy, many observers dismissed the voice channel of telephone communication, assuming that most of it would be displaced by digital data. However, as with digital radiology, the combination of a powerful new industry data standard, VoiceXML, and sophisticated speech-recognition software promise to revolutionize and personalize voice communication, both for users and for firms with large, telephone-connected customer bases.[34]

Eliza Corporation, whose technology was initially developed at California Institute of Technology, builds voice-response software that enables caregivers, health plans, and disease management companies to interact with patients at home. The software algorithm at the heart of Eliza is so sophisticated that it can recognize and respond to millions of responses to the question, "Is this Jeff Goldsmith?" including coughing, handing the phone to someone else, and responses in other languages. Eliza is so warm and accepting that patients or family members will reliably return its calls if they are not at home to receive the initial call.[35]

Computerized voice-response technologies will help lift the burden of care and worry from family members of elderly or chronically ill patients who need reminders to take their medications, periodic updates on their condition, appointment reminders or patient education and outreach, such as mammogram or vaccination reminders.

THE INTERNET: A REVOLUTION IN CONNECTIVITY

Technology experts might quibble about whether the Internet is not so much a technology as a remarkably flexible and expandable communications platform for a host of new technologies. However, no one would quarrel with the assertion that no technology since the invention of the telephone has created such a sensation as the Internet.

The Internet enabled instantaneous and asynchronous communication between any parties connected at first to an existing telephone network and later using cable, ground-based wireless, and satellite modalities, allowing the Internet to be accessed in automobiles, airplanes, or literally anywhere in the world where one can receive a wireless signal. With increased bandwidth has come the ability to transmit virtually any form of digital information, including sound and both still and streaming video files.

People who use the Internet are on a mission; they actively use the Internet to seek knowledge and connection to others. The Internet is the mother of all knowledge management and communication tools. Society seemed to awaken in the mid-1990s to discover that it had grown a whole new nervous system. The connections spawned by the Internet have resulted in the spontaneous formation of what futurist Howard Rheingold dubbed "virtual communities" revolving around common interests and issues.[36]

The Internet and Health Information

Health-related information was among the most immediately popular points of convergence. Six million people use the Internet to seek health information every day, just in the United States,[37] and according to the Pew Trust Internet American Life Project, 62 percent of adults connected to the Internet sought health information through it.[38] The Internet became a vehicle by which consumers learned to bypass the traditional sources of medical information—physicians—and connect directly to journal and research articles and to other patients or family members coping with a given disease. Internet applications have empowered consumers to define their own medical reality and to reframe and broaden their relationships to physicians.

The Internet and Health Plans

As discussed in Chapter 6, the Internet has also brought a host of powerful new applications to health plans to communicate with their vast and diffuse networks of subscribers, corporate customers, and the health system itself. These applications form the core of an emerging "consumer directed" model of health insurance.[39] The most exciting healthcare applications of Internet technology may be found in the health insurance arena.

The Internet and Healthcare Delivery

Internet applications have less direct saliency to hospitals and other healthcare delivery institutions, where improving clinical and financial operations is the most immediate management challenge. However, Internet technologies will be used to make hospitals and the information they contain more accessible to patients and families.[40] Furthermore, because the Internet dissolves organizational boundaries, not only in medicine but in every other part of our economy, it will eventually enable the unbundling and outsourcing of many core hospital administrative functions, such as finance and IT management, which have challenged healthcare managers for years. The Internet will enable the birth of a huge new industy of business process outsourcing in healthcare.

Overall Effects of the Internet on Healthcare

What the Internet has provided is affordable and nearly universal connectivity, enabling physicians and consumers to connect to one another and to the rest of the health system through their existing communications channels, such as the telephone line or cable. By democratizing connectivity, the Internet has brought the health system and its users closer together.

The Internet has also provided a new communications backbone to speed transactions and reduce clerical expenses in the vast bureaucratic sprawl that the American health system has become. As discussed earlier in this chapter, it has also provided a readily usable platform for projecting clinical information across different care sites. One way to think about the Internet is as a technology enabler or, in military jargon, a force multiplier, that helps lower communications and transaction cost, time, and complexity. It is also a lubricant of information flow and a solvent of organizational boundaries. It may take at least another decade before the health system realizes the full extent of its transformative potential.

Sadly, in healthcare, nothing happens on "Internet time."

THE ELECTRONIC MEDICAL RECORD: THE POINT OF CONVERGENCE

Digital technologies have vastly expanded the accuracy and geographical reach of medical care and enabled earlier and timelier intervention in disease processes. However, the reason why digitizing vital health information is important is that it enables this information to be assembled electronically and directed to the point of medical decisions.

The single point of convergence of all this digital information about health—genetic disease risk and vulnerability to therapy; the genetic signatures of viruses, bacteria, and tumor cells; the digital images of internal organs (structure and metabolic function); the current state of physical health from sensors outside the body and devices inside it; health history; and the record of what drugs and therapies have been prescribed—is the so-called "electronic medical record" (EMR) (Figure 2.4).

Early Generations of EMRs

Hospitals began experimenting with digitizing patient information in the early 1970s with mixed results. Early experimenters included academic health centers like the University of Indiana and Boston's Brigham and Women's Hospital and multihospital systems like Utah's Intermountain Health Care. These early efforts involved creating a clinical data repository into which medical record information was entered for later retrieval and analysis. As new in-

Figure 2.4: Digital Medicine: Converging Streams

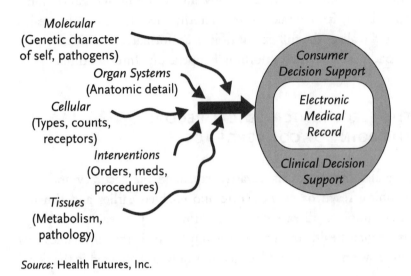

Molecular
(Genetic character
of self, pathogens)

Organ Systems
(Anatomic detail)

Cellular
(Types, counts,
receptors)

Interventions
(Orders, meds,
procedures)

Tissues
(Metabolism,
pathology)

*Consumer
Decision Support*

*Electronic
Medical
Record*

*Clinical Decision
Support*

Source: Health Futures, Inc.

formation was generated about the patient's condition or orders or prescriptions are written for him or her, this new information was entered into the repository. Physicians and other caregivers could then enter orders electronically and get test results and other clinical data on their patients.

However, data storage and database management technologies were so primitive, and computing power so modest, that it was extremely cumbersome for physicians to retrieve information at the point of care (e.g., the patient bed, the operating suite, the ICU, etc.). Until the advent of the Apple Macintosh and, later, the Windows operating system in the mid-1980s, physicians who wanted to undertake computerized physician order entry had to learn an awkward language of computer commands and type those commands into the computer to manage their patients or to retrieve or use clinical information.

As will be seen in Chapter 3, these efforts were also hampered by the highly fragmented record structure of hospitals. Hospitals have historically maintained separate record systems in each clinical department (for the laboratory, the operating room, the radiology department, the emergency room, etc.). These so-called "legacy" systems were constructed primarily for billing purposes, not for care management. Legacy clinical systems are like a gigantic tangle of weedy undergrowth that strangles the care process as well as the efforts of those nurses, physicians, and other caregivers who use them.

Even small hospitals may have as many as two dozen legacy clinical information systems. Unbelievably, large health systems with multiple hospitals may have as many as 500 legacy systems, purchased from different vendors, written in different software languages, and operating on different, often incompatible hardware. These systems can be made to "interoperate" (i.e., move information across systems electronically) only by writing expensive custom software interfaces to link them or, more recently, with expensive "web services" that perform the same functions over the Internet.

As a consequence of this tangle, slightly different versions of our clinical reality exist in as many as 15 different places inside the hospital. The fact that there is no unified picture of an individual's health status is a hazard to that person's health. Creating a unified repository of all information requires a common format for clinical information, a single patient identifier applied across departments, and an agreement by all those who provide care to contribute what they know to the digital record.

Interactive Clinical Information Systems

Even where this unified repository was achieved, the early generations of EMRs were little more than digital versions of the patient's chart, that is, a jumbled, historical compilation of what has been done to a patient. In the early 1980s, this began to change as the result of a collaboration between Intermountain Health Care and the

3M Corporation produced the first interactive clinical information system, called HELP.

HELP was the UNIVAC of intelligent clinical information systems. (I saw it demonstrated in 1983 at 3M's headquarters in Minneapolis and was appropriately dazzled.) This system evaluated medication orders, compared them to the known medications patients were using and their current condition, and alerted the clinical team to potential problems. HELP also recorded whether the clinical team had read the alert and required them to override the system to proceed with ordering the treatment.

Clinical Decision Support

Clinical decision support played an increasingly prominent role in emerging clinical systems. In the mid-1980s, intensive care specialists at George Washington University led by Dr. William Knaus built an "intelligent" clinical system called APACHE to forecast patient outcomes in the intensive care unit and help the clinical team predict more accurately whether patients were going to survive. APACHE represented a significant advance because it added a predictive dimension to clinical decision support and guided, rather than passively alerting, care decision makers.

Intelligent Clinical Management Software

HELP and APACHE were the forerunners of a new type of clinical information system being developed by commercial vendors. Today, creators of clinical management software, including Cerner, Siemens, General Electric, Epic, Eclipsys, and IDX, are all working toward creating a seamless care management toolset undergirded by decision support that can follow patients across an episode of care.

This emerging intelligent clinical management software technology is at the forefront of healthcare IT development and represents the leading edge of a societal investment that could exceed $100 billion over the next decade in the United States alone. Altogether, these tools may be the most complex commercial software products ever built, considering that they are automating what may be the most complex process in the economy—health service.

A NAVIGATION SYSTEM FOR CLINICAL CARE

To describe this merger of the digital patient record with decision support as a "medical record" does not do justice to the innovation. Clinical systems are becoming "context aware," meaning that they will be wired to diagnostic devices and patient monitoring equipment. They can track real-time changes in the patient's health and will follow patients as they move through different levels of care—from an ambulatory diagnosis through surgery, into recovery, or even into home healthcare. These new systems now alert care providers when the patient's condition changes, prompting the clinical team to take specific actions to deal with an emerging problem.

Most importantly, however, clinical systems are reaching a sufficient level of intelligence to bring up-to-date medical knowledge to the physician's office, exam room, or hospital bed. As medical science better defines how to treat patients, that knowledge will flow through computer systems to the point of care. The clinical system will prompt physicians, nurses, and others involved in patient care to follow the care pathway that holds the most promise for improving the patient's health.

The Clinician's Role

These systems do not relieve physicians and the care team of their professional and moral obligation in making patient care decisions. Just as those who use a navigational system in an airplane have the ultimate responsibility for reaching the destination safely, the clinical team is going to remain accountable—to patients, family members, colleagues, the courts, and society—for making the right decisions. However, clinical decision support is transforming the electronic medical record into a powerful advocate for patient safety, as well as a research tool for recording and investigating what works in medicine (Figure 2.5).

Physicians who want to understand the basis for the system's recommendations will be able to look behind the recommendations to the research studies and clinical drug trial results and even review the outcomes of care for the last several hundred patients who received a particular treatment in the hospital to see what clinical strategies have worked best.

The traditional medical record documents a patient's health history and any treatments provided. The clinical information systems presented here will be more like navigational systems in an airliner. Harris Berman, a physician who founded the Tufts Health Plan in New England, described this clinical system in a speech made in April 2002 to a group of colleagues at the Gartner Healthcare IT Summit in Boston, characterizing it as a medical version of the NeverLost (the trademarked global positioning system Hertz uses in its rental cars). It will locate the patient in the sphere of medical risk, constantly update the clinical team on his or her condition, and indicate a trajectory based on the latest scientific knowledge to help the care team negotiate the patient through an episode of care.

BEYOND THE NAVIGATION SYSTEM TO TEACHER/KNOWLEDGE ORGANIZER

As decision support becomes richer and more flexible, clinical systems will evolve a step further, into a powerful knowledge management tool that continuously teaches the clinical team about the changing state of medical knowledge. It will also serve as a powerful

Figure 2.5: Evolution of the "EMR"

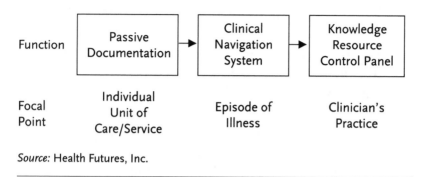

Function	Passive Documentation	→	Clinical Navigation System	→	Knowledge Resource Control Panel
Focal Point	Individual Unit of Care/Service		Episode of Illness		Clinician's Practice

Source: Health Futures, Inc.

care manager to reach, monitor, and safeguard patients who are no longer hospitalized nor even under the physician's direct care.

The system will present a clinical "dashboard" to the physician each morning, in whatever form and venue he or she chooses (home or office desktop, portable laptop or tablet computer, or personal digital assistant). Clinical systems will be intelligent enough to recognize their users by their past inquiries and even their different cognitive styles. This latter capability is especially helpful, because physicians do not all think about a medical problem the same way. Most physicians will bridle against a rigid, prepackaged approach to making care decisions. As clinical systems evolve, they will be able to recognize those cognitive differences and enable physicians or other caregivers to acquire and process information in a way with which they are comfortable.

With the advent of XML, the Internet tagging convention, and powerful new search engines, clinical information systems will also be able to reach out and identify new medical knowledge of interest for their clinical users or for patients and family members. Moreover, using past search criteria (much as Amazon.com does today for purchasers of books and compact discs), clinical systems will be able to identify new knowledge—research papers, results of clinical trials, new drugs and new indications for existing drugs, for example—

that fits the clinician's search patterns and "push" it to his or her dashboard automatically.

Clinical software will enable physicians to stratify their patients, active and inactive, into risk groups and will both organize and maintain communication with them to ensure not only that their inquiries are answered, but also that they are complying with treatment recommendations. It will "remember" prescriptions and communicate with patients or family members about whether the therapy is producing the desired results. Clinical software will automatically schedule follow-up appointments and send patients information electronically on their illness and treatment options. Information systems will also link them automatically to disease management programs, managed by voice-response tools such as Eliza, to interact with patients to ensure that they are taking their medications as prescribed and managing their own health effectively.

The remote patient monitoring systems discussed earlier, whether they are wearable devices like the wireless cardiac monitor, passive sensors like those used in the smart house, or implantable devices like Medtronic's intelligent pacemakers, will connect "patients" to physicians or the care team through their clinical information systems. (Indeed, we are straining the term "patient" here, as many who will be monitored and protected by these systems are not, strictly speaking, ill, but rather at risk. We need a new term for people at medical risk that does not imply that they are institutionalized or under active care.) The initial layer of monitoring will be done by the computer system itself, sending alerts to physicians, nurses, or family members through wireless Internet connections if something threatens the patient's health.

TECHNICAL CONSTRAINTS

Standing between us and the achievement of this vision are several important technical constraints.

The Evolving State of Medical Knowledge

The most significant challenge is the evolving state of medical knowledge. Until very recently, medical science has been remarkably incurious about what treatments actually improve the patient's health. Safety, not efficacy, has been the principal focus both of research and of regulation. With the advent of what is now known as the Agency for Health Research and Quality in the Department of Health and Human Services, the federal government in 1989 began funding research into clinical outcomes. Additionally, more than 180 organizations, including medical and surgical specialty societies, academic health centers, and commercial companies, are developing scientifically based clinical guidelines.[41] This emerging knowledge base is critical to the "intelligence" as well as the scope of clinical software.

Natural Language Processing

Another important constraint is the interface with the clinician. Although moving from typing to pointing and clicking helped make clinical software more accessible, the ability of clinicians to enter new information and interact with the system still depends more than it ought to on a mouse or keypad. Physicians do not like to type; they are used to dictating (and correcting, and reviewing, and correcting again). Removing typing or pointing and clicking from the process of interacting with the clinical system will require advances not in speech recognition, which is surprisingly powerful today, but in something called "natural language processing."

Natural language processing will not only be used to allow software to communicate with patients over the phone, but it will also enable a computer system to understand what a clinician means when he or she describes a clinical condition. It depends on a "controlled medical vocabulary," which recognizes that terms like "heart attack," "myocardial infarction," "acute MI," and so on, all refer to the same condition. Prying common meanings loose from the stream of words recognized by a computer system is the technical challenge that stands between today's clinical systems that rely on typing or point-and-click interfaces and a truly interactive voice-response capability. According to Gartner, a respected technology evaluation firm, this capability may still be a decade off.[42]

Improving the Graphical User Interface

The graphical user interface, or GUI—that is, the shape and configuration that the system presents to its user—also represents a significant constraint. Most clinical GUIs are based on some version of the Windows system and are overly busy, unattractive, and user-unfriendly. How to present clinical information and treatment options in a way that clinicians find accessible and easy to use is a less visible, but very significant, barrier to adoption by clinicians.

The "desktop" may not be the best visual metaphor to use in organizing this information. David Gelernter, a brilliant computer scientist, has proposed a chronological stream or ordering of ideas or documents by the time they first connected to the user as an alternative to the more static idea of a desktop.[43] Advances in human engineering will be required to make clinical systems more transparent and easier to adapt to clinical use.

Stabilizing and Strengthening Wireless Technology

Many clinicians want to be able to practice medicine from anywhere and not be chained to a computer terminal in their offices or the hospital. A surprisingly large percentage of physicians (26 percent as of 2001) and virtually all medical students and residents in training own personal digital assistants.[44] The ability to practice medicine from anywhere is constrained by the inability thus far to create secure wireless networks for clinical information with sufficient bandwidth and robustness to transmit bulky, complex medical files. As anyone who owns a cell phone knows, wireless technology is still a fragile, frustrating, and insecure medium.

Hospital structures in particular are exceptionally hostile environments for wireless technology, with lead shielding, structural steel, elevators, and an almost lethal amount of radio frequency signals from myriad devices and conduits. "Practicing from anywhere" will require more powerful devices, improved (and probably larger) device screens, increased security, and the installation of wireless infrastructure in hospitals, clinics, and physicians' offices. This may take the better part of a decade as well.

Nontechnical Issues

Two nontechnical constraints will be more fully discussed in the chapters that follow. They are (1) high cost, a major challenge for hospitals, health plans, physicians, and everyone else in the health system, and (2) the need to rethink and reorganize the care process and culture of medical practice itself, which may be the most daunting challenge of all. The balance of this book will discuss the nature of these constraints and how they may be overcome.

Despite these challenges, IT is on the verge of revolutionizing how medicine is practiced and how consumers and patients experience it. It will reduce the barriers to communication within the clinical team by reducing the need for face-to-face or simultaneous use of communication tools like the telephone and enable medicine to be practiced on, literally, a global scale. It will also tighten the links between the clinical team and the patient and liberate both from what Don Berwick has termed "the tyranny of the visit."

Thanks to IT, medicine's safety net will broaden to literally anywhere and be woven unobtrusively into the fabric of life. With computer assistance, medicine will become not only more virtual, but more intelligent and safer. Digital medicine is responsive, personalized medicine—anywhere, anytime. The next four chapters discuss how these technologies will affect the major actors in the American healthcare system.

NOTES

1. Ridley, M. 1999. *Genome*. New York: HarpersCollins Publishers, Inc.

2. Neaves, W., president, Stowers Institute for Genetic Research. Personal communication, April 2001.

3. Reuters Business Insight. 2002. *The Genomics Outlook to 2005: Transforming Pharmaceutical and Diagnostic Markets. Healthcare Report*. London: Reuters Business Insight.

4. Burrill, S. 2002. *Biotech 2002: Life Sciences: Systems Biology*. The Biotechnology Industry 16th Annual Report. San Francisco: Burrill and Company.

5. Hirsch, M. S., B. Conway, R. T. D'Aquila, V. A. Johnson, F. Brun-Vézinet, B. Clotet, L. M. Demeter, S. M. Hammer, D. M. Jacobsen, D. R. Kuritzkes, C. Loveday, J. W. Mellors, S. Vella, and D. D. Richman. 1998. "Antiretroviral Drug Resistance Testing in Adults with HIV Infection." *Journal of the American Medical Association* 279 (4): 1984–91.

6. Lazarou, J., B. H. Pomeranz, and P. N. Corey. 1998. "Incidence of Adverse Drug Reactions in Hospitalized Patients: A Meta-analysis of Prospective Studies." *Journal of the American Medical Association* 279 (15): 1200–05.

7. Phillips, K. A., D. L. Veenstra, E. Oren, J. K. Lee, and W. Sadee. 2001. "Potential Role of Pharmacogenomics in Reducing Adverse Drug Reactions: A Systematic Review." *Journal of the American Medical Association* 286 (18): 2270–79.

8. Ibid. Burrill, S. 2002.

9. Groopman, J. 1998. "Dr. Fair's Tumor." *The New Yorker* Oct. 26, 78–106.

10. Arnst, C. 2001. "New Cancer Weapons Strut Their Stuff." *Business Week Online* May 10. [Online article; retrieved 11/20/02.] Boulder, CO: Business Week. http://www.businessweek.com/technology/content/may2001/tc20010510_835.htm.

11. Carmichael, G. G. 2002. "Silencing Viruses with RNA." *Nature* 418: 379–80.

12. Burrill, S. 2001. *Biotech 2001: Life Sciences: Genomics, Proteonomics . . . and More*. The Biotechnology Industry 15th Annual Report. San Francisco: Burrill and Company.

13. GE Medical Systems. 2001. "GE Medical Systems Unveils Breakthrough Technology to Aid Doctors in Early Detection and Diagnosis of Cancer." [Online

press release; retrieved 1/2/03.] http://apps.gemedicalsystems.com/apps3/pressroom/news_release_detail.jsp?A=false&RECID=211681.

14. Hackworth, M. 1999. "Now, Software Must Take Over: Even If Chips No Longer Follow Moore's Law, Efficiencies Don't Have to End." *San Jose Mercury News,* Oct. 19.

15. Greenes, R. A., and J. F. Brinkley. 2001. "Imaging Systems." In *Medical Informatics: Computer Application in Health Care and Biomedicine,* edited by E. H. Shortliffe and L. E. Perreault, 485–538. New York: Springer Verlag.

16. Hammond, W. E., and J. J. Cimino. 2001. "Standards in Medical Informatics." In *Medical Informatics: Computer Application in Health Care and Biomedicine,* edited by E. H. Shortliffe and L. E. Perreault, 212–56. New York: Springer Verlag.

17. Philips, D. 2002. Interview with associate chair, Radiology Department, University of Virginia.

18. Freer, T. W., and M. J. Ulissey. 2001. "Screening Mammography with Computer-aided Detection: Prospective Study of 12,860 Patients in a Community Breast Center." *Radiology* 220 (3): 781–86.

19. David, D., and E. L. Michelson. 1988. "Transtelephonic Electrocardiographic Monitoring for the Detection and Treatment of Cardiac Arrhythmias." *Cardiovascular Clinics* 18 (3): 73–82.

20. Antman, E. M., P. L. Ludmer, N. McGowan, M. Bosak, and P. L. Friedman. 1986. "Transtelephonic Electrocardiographic Transmission for Management of Cardiac Arrhythmias." *American Journal of Cardiology* 58 (10): 1021–24.

21. Ginsburg, R., I. H. Lamb, J. S. Schroeder, and D. C. Harrison. 1981. "Long-term Transtelephonic Electrocardiographic Monitoring in the Detection and Evaluation of Variant Angina." *American Heart Journal* 102 (2): 196–201.

22. CardioNet. 2002. "CardioNet Closes $18.5 Million Financing Round." [Online press release; retrieved 1/2/03]. Philadelphia, PA: CardioNet. http://www.cardionet.com/pr_03_09_02.html.

23. Becker, C. 2002. "Remote Control." *Modern Healthcare.* [Online information; retrieved 12/14/02.] Chicago: Crain Communications, Inc. http://www.modernhealthcare.com/article.cms?articleId=1712.

24. Becker, C. 2001. "Telemedicine System Helps Manage ICUs." *Modern Healthcare.* [Online information; retrieved 12/14/02.] Chicago: Crain Communications, Inc. http://www.modernhealthcare.com/article.cms?articleId=5148.

25. Medtronic. 1999. "Medtronic Launches World's Smallest Implantable, Single Chamber Defibrillator with Rate-responsive Pacing." [Online press release; retrieved 1/2/03.] Minneapolis, MN: Medtronic. http://www.medtronic.com/newsroom/news_release.html#HTML.

26. Dunn., J. 2003. "A Physician with a Dash of Engineer." *New York Times*, Jan. 5.

27. Medtronic. 2003. "Medtronic's New Hand-Held Programmer for Neurological Therapies Gives Clinicians More Features and 'Palm-Sized Convenience.'" [Online press release; retrieved 1/7/03.] Minneapolis, MN: Medtronic. http://www.medtronic.com/newsroom/news_20030107a.html.

28. Felder, R. A., S. Graves, and T. Mifflin. 1999. "Reading the Future: The Increased Relevance of Laboratory Medicine in the Next Century." *Medical Laboratory Observer* 31 (7): 20–1, 24–6.

29. Eisenberg, A. 2001. "A 'Smart' Home, to Avoid the Nursing Home." *New York Times*, April 5.

30. Berck, J. 2001. "The Wired Retirement Home." *New York Times*, April 5.

31. Marescaux, J., J. Leroy, M. Gagner, F. Rubino, D. Mutter, M. Vix, S. E. Butner, and M. K. Smith. 2001. "Transatlantic Robot-assisted Surgery." *Nature* 413: 379–80.

32. National Library of Medicine. 2002. "The Visible Human Project." [Online information; retrieved 12/2/02.] Bethesda, MD: National Library of Medicine. http://www.nlm.nih.gov/research/visible/visible_human.html.

33. Mitka, M. 2001. "US Military Medicine Moves to Meet Current Challenge." *Journal of the American Medical Association* 286 (20): 2532–33.

34. "The Power of Voice." 2002. *The Economist Technology Quarterly*. [Online article; retrieved 1/4/03]. http://www.economist.com/printedition/displayStory.cfm?Story_ID=1476779.

35. Merrow, L. 2002. Interview with chief executive officer, Eliza Corporation, December 23.

36. Rheingold, H. 2000. *Virtual Community: Homesteading on the Electronic Frontier 2000*. Cambridge, MA: MIT Press.

37. T. Ferguson. 2002. "e-Patients, Online Health, and the Search for Sustainable Healthcare: A Guide for Grantmakers." Working Paper. Princeton, NJ: The Robert Wood Johnson Foundation.

38. Fox, S., and L. Rainie. 2000. "The Online Healthcare Revolution: How the Web is Helping Americans Take Better Care of Themselves." Washington, DC: Pew Trust Internet American Life Project.

39. Goldsmith, J. C. 2000. "The Internet and Managed Care: A New Wave of Innovation." *Health Affairs* 19 (6): 42–56.

40. Goldsmith, J. C. 2001. "How Hospitals Should Be Using the Internet." *Internet Healthcare Strategies* 3 (1): 1–4.

41. Meaney, B., and G. Belfiglio. 2002. "Putting Clinical Guidelines to Work." *Medicine on the Net* 8 (3): 1–4.

42. Gartner, Inc. 2001. "Strategic Technology Planning." In *eHealthcare Summit 2001: Separating Reality From Fantasy*. Stamford, CT: Gartner.

43. Abreu, E. 2001. "There Has To Be a Better Way." *The Industry Standard*. [Online article; retrieved 12/20/02.] Boston: IDG. http://www.thestandard.com/article /0,1902,23643,00.html?body_page=1.

44. Taylor, H., and R. Leitman, eds. 2001. "Physicians' Use of Handheld Personal Computing Devices Increases from 15 percent in 1999 to 26 percent in 2001." *Harris Interactive* 1 (25): 1–4.

CHAPTER 3

Hospitals

LIKE STEEL MILLS and department stores, hospitals are creatures of the "old economy." As primitive knowledge "machines," hospitals have historically relied on bringing together diverse health professionals in the same physical location to coalesce around solving our complex health problems. As Rosemary Stevens has written in her marvelous history, *In Sickness and in Wealth*, American hospitals have proved to be remarkably adept at co-opting new technologies (surgery and anesthesia, to name only two examples) to change their business.[1]

Although I cast doubt on their ability to continue this successful adaptation in a 1981 book entitled *Can Hospitals Survive?*, the ensuing sextupling of revenues (from $70 billion in 1978 to $451 billion in 2001) speaks to this institution's impressive economic and social power.[2] Despite a host of new, portable medical technologies (like noninvasive imaging and fiberoptic scopes) and an array of serious challenges during the past decade from health plans and physician group practice, hospitals remain today at the center of the U.S. health system.

Hospitals stand on the cusp of an information revolution that will profoundly alter their operations and culture and markedly improve the safety of their services. Hospitals have struggled for the past decade with immature technologies, troubled vendor relationships, and overtaxed information technology staff to cope with what may be the most complex computing challenge in the entire economy. To take advantage of current and emerging technologies, hospitals will have to leap forward 20 years from an information architecture still sadly dependent on paper and the telephone.

A BRIEF, SAD HISTORY OF HOSPITAL COMPUTING

The information architecture of most contemporary hospitals is like a 1950s metropolis built on top of an ancient Roman city, the street grid and much of the water and sewer infrastructure "inherited" from an earlier historical era. Hospitals and other health systems spent an estimated $20 billion acquiring and installing IT in the year 2000.[3] This spending rests on a rotting foundation, however, and a depressing fraction is spent on maintenance of the foundation rather than on innovation.

Unless one is building a completely new hospital from scratch in a "green field," as hospital developers call it, IT solutions must build on the legacy information systems hospitals already have in place. Importantly, these legacy systems constrain the ability of any new computer installation to work properly because any new system has to "interface" with many of the old systems.

Hospitals began trying to computerize their business functions during the 1960s. Computerization began with hospital departments partially automating their operations one at a time. The process began with billing and accounting functions and radiated out into the major revenue-generating clinical departments (clinical laboratory, pharmacy, radiology, etc.). Computerization focused on assembling the information needed to bill for the hospital's diverse clinical services. This department-by-department approach is sometimes called "functional computing," as each function demanded and got its own computer system.*

The Slippery Slope to Babel

As minicomputers began appearing in the early 1980s, hospitals took the inevitable step toward distributed computing. Minicomputers, followed rapidly by personal computers, made department-based functional computing suddenly affordable. Hospitals began acquiring minicomputers, and then personal computers and servers, by the freight-car load.

Reinforcing Fragmentation

Viewed from the safety of 20 years' hindsight, the PC era of hospital computing was a giant step backward for patients and society. This is because the easy availability of systems based on personal computers and small servers reinforced the fragmentation of the hospital itself. Each profession or technical function in the hospital has its own department (a large hospital may have as many as 80 departments). Each profession also has its own unique view of its centrality to the patient care process, its own ideology and language system, and, thanks to the PC, its own information system.

---

*Ironically, the earliest hospital business computing applications were network models. Mainframe computers were so expensive that almost no hospital could afford its own. So it made economic sense for hospitals to employ a time-sharing, remote computing model. As time-sharing on commercial mainframe computers became widely available, hospital IT firms such as Shared Medical Systems (SMS, now part of Siemens) developed departmental applications and made them available through modem connections to their remote processing centers. The fact that tomorrow's computer systems will employ a network model recapitulates the first 15 years of hospital computing history.

In theory, all these professionals work together both in patient care and in supporting administrative activities. In practical reality, in many hospitals, collaboration between professional departments is grudging at best. Through the clinical and support departments they control, professions in the hospital compete for resources and control over patients. Furthermore, physicians, who control where patients are cared for, are increasingly directing patients with less complex illnesses to settings they control, like surgi-centers and freestanding heart hospitals. The boundaries separating the hospital from other caregivers are constantly shifting, due in major part to economic incentives and other nonclinical factors.

Internal competition among hospital departments and the need to compete with freestanding facilities (like surgi-centers and heart hospitals, many of which have physician investors) results in an unseemly clamor for capital spending. Allocating capital dollars between facilities and equipment (the traditional uses of capital) and IT (the emerging use of capital) is a political and managerial nightmare for hospital managements and trustees.[4]

The Private-Practice Physician Imposes an Additional Constraint

Most American physicians are administratively independent of the hospitals whose clinical activities they direct. Physicians who *are* employees (and one-third are employed by someone, according to American Medical Association data) tend to be employed by physician-dominated entities (group practices, academic faculty practice plans), which are organizationally distinct from the hospital.[5]

The reason this is a problem from an information technology standpoint is that physicians maintain separate records in their offices or clinics, which do not link to the hospital's record on the same patient. Because 83 percent of physicians' records are in paper form, building interfaces from the hospital or other physicians' offices to reach them is technically impossible.[6] Pre- and post-hospital care under the physician's oversight is in a different information and management domain than care rendered in the hospital. The hospital-physician clinical information boundary is like the blood-brain barrier in the body—a virtually impermeable boundary that traps information on either side that is needed to render safe healthcare.

For all these reasons, short of running a large urban school system, running a hospital may be one of the most demanding and frustrating jobs in the entire economy. Given all the battles hospital executives have to fight, it has been easier historically to dole out IT willy-nilly on a department-by-department basis than to insist on orderly collaboration and shared systems. Hospital chief information officers (CIOs) often despair of functioning more as traffic cops than planners, mediating disputes over resources, timing, and systems compatibility. In the political wheeling and dealing, often the vision of a future information architecture that works for patients and physicians gets lost in the struggle to accommodate the historical culture of the hospital and to meet the short-term needs of its departments.

Fragmentation Affects Patients

Departmental records were not organized primarily to support or coordinate patient care, which inevitably involves multiple departments. Rather, departmental record-keeping systems were created to support billing for the department's services. Each department had its own registration and scheduling function; each departmental system assigned the patient a different identification number.

This is why, until very recently, a multidepartment hospital visit required a patient to re-register at each stop. In each location, clerks handed patients clipboards with forms that asked questions such as their social security number, mother's maiden name, and health history. Each time they visited, patients were asked for the same information yet again, as if they were strangers. In many cases, the information was inaccessible in a physician's office and needed to be duplicated in the hospital. In this fragmented information world, crucial information (like what drugs patients are allergic to, what happened the last time they were hospitalized, or what their blood type is) often was very difficult to obtain at the moment in time in which patients were in the office to influence and guide their care.

To address this problem, hospitals had to purchase a software product called the Enterprise Master Patient Index (EMPI), which traces every individual patient's records in the different departments and matches them up so the system can "pretend" that they are actually the same person in all those different places. In a medium-sized hospital, it cost upwards of $500,000 just to install an EMPI program.

Moreover, if the hospital wants the dozen or more separate patient records for each patient to actually come together, it must hire a consulting firm to provide "systems integration." This has been a spectacular and lucrative consulting franchise because systems integration is *endless*. Each time the hospital adds a new computer system, someone must write custom software code to get the new system to talk to the other, older systems.

ENTERPRISE COMPUTING

It seems like an obvious solution to have a single, enterprisewide information architecture and a unified, manageable flow of clinical information to those who need it. In enterprisewide computing, the hospital has a single (digital) clinical record, a single patient identifier that every department and professional uses, a common repository for clinical and financial information, and an ability to retrieve that information quickly anywhere in the organization that it is needed.

The problem is that replacing all the information systems in a hospital is costly and painful. As J. D. Kleinke wrote in an oft-quoted 1998 analysis, enterprise software in hospitals has been a costly disappointment for most institutions.[7] Kleinke blames the "hype cycle" and the pervasive economic incentive for vendors to foist "vaporware" on customers. Certainly this has been a real (and continuing) problem—vendors promising complex applications that are not completed.

However, I believe the problem is larger than the reality of how hard it is to build complex tools that work. The fact that it has been so difficult to automate what hospitals do reflects the almost crippling complexity of what hospitals do and, indeed, what they are. Healthcare is the most complex thing our economy produces; there is more variability and uncertainty at the point of care in an emergency room, intensive care unit, or hospital operating suite than in just about any other part of our economy.

Furthermore, there is no "operating manual." A physician cannot just turn to a "standard operating procedure" in a given clinical circumstance (although he or she will be able to for many illnesses or conditions in about ten more years). The "answer" is supposed to be in the physician's head. That is what their training and professional culture told them.

However, the fundamental reason why enterprise computing has been so difficult to implement in hospitals is that many of them are not really enterprises. This is the real reason they are so hard to manage. They *look* like enterprises, with buildings, budgets, and organizational charts, but they function more like loose collections of professions uncomfortably housed in the same physical structures. A coral reef is such a structure, much more a colorful Darwinian ecology than a sentient being.

Information systems are like nervous systems. The nervous system for a jellyfish is going to look and function differently than the nervous system for a higher, thinking organism. Hospitals are like large amoeboid organisms with poorly developed central nervous systems. The organism, as much as the wiring, is the constraint. One can design a nervous system for a collaborative enterprise, but one should not be surprised if it does not work very well if the actors in the enterprise really do not effectively collaborate. There is no functional substitute for a "brain," or for teamwork.

In addition to the physiology of the organism, there is a work-force problem. Until very recently, health executive and professional education ignored information technology. Most knowledge about IT is acquired "on the street" rather than in the classroom. Because IT has been so hard to acquire and use, most of the street experience has not been all that helpful—how to circumvent the system to get what you want or how to build shadow paper-and-telephone networks to support day-to-day activity.

There is a critical shortage of technically trained, competent workers in every sector of healthcare IT. Vendors as well as providers struggle to find qualified workers at every skill level. Since what they collectively do—install and operate information systems—is somewhat akin to rewiring an automobile while it is running, it should not be surprising to learn that IT workers burn out quickly.

Clinical Quality and Decision Support

The previous chapter describes the promise of the intelligent clinical information system, undergirded by clinical decision support and care guidelines. The increasing intelligence of clinical information systems has the potential for markedly reducing medical errors.[8] This is not only because those systems can ensure that physicians make decisions based on timely and accurate information, but because they also computerize the decision-making process (computerizing physician and nursing orders) itself, reducing the delays and uncertainties produced by written (and often illegible) prescriptions, test results, and care orders. Rules engines built into clinical software will examine the orders themselves to ensure that they are what the physician or nurse intended, compare them to what is known about the patient's present condition, and provide a "reality" check on care decisions automatically.

The central challenge these new clinical tools pose to hospital managements is that they fundamentally challenge the fragmentation of the hospital experience—and an operating culture that places the needs of hospital departments and professions above the needs of the patient. IT vendors experience this frustration in installing new clinical systems because they are effectively asked to digitize every existing care process in the hospital. Instead, hospital leaders should collaborate with the IT community to redesign how care is rendered to make it seamless to the patient, to improve communication within the care team, and to provide accountability for making care safer and more efficient.

Realistically, however, sophisticated IT by itself will not reduce medical errors. Computer systems could help alleviate, but are not going to eliminate, professional burnout, poor morale, rivalries among professional groups, continuity problems between clinical departments ("it's not my department; she's not my patient"), and the potential for "dropped batons" in a complex hospitalization.

Thoughtfully designed computer systems can make the practice of medicine much easier, but in the final analysis, how effectively the right decisions are made ultimately determines whether patients are safe. Until clinical care becomes truly team based and an ethos of "how would I want my loved one treated here?" pervades patient floors, exam rooms, and surgical suites, a lot of unacceptable risk will remain in the care system, regardless of the capability of the computer system. Information systems will not absolve clinicians of their moral and professional responsibilities to make thoughtful decisions in the patient's interests.

In other words, changing the culture of healthcare is something we cannot rely on technology alone to accomplish. Capital spending is no substitute for compassion, patient-centered values, and, most of all, leadership. Absent the leadership, all the expensive tools in the world are not going to be used to the ultimate benefit of the patient and society.

CONNECTING THE HOSPITAL

Network computing returned to the hospital world around 1998, engulfed in a tornado of hype. The Internet was going to revolutionize healthcare IT, enabling hospitals and other healthcare organizations to circumvent all the complexities discussed above and simply move information freely and quickly to where it was needed.

One medical informatics pioneer, Clem McDonald, offered the metaphor of network computing as a rain forest canopy, where arboreal creatures (presumably physicians) could move effortlessly across the canopy picking fruit (clinical information) without the need to climb all of the individual trees.[9]

Of course, how the fruit grows in the canopy is one of those mysteries of nature. Clearly, nutrients and water have to reach the fruit from somewhere. How does all that clinical information get onto the Internet in the first place? One has to wade into all those messy departmental systems (emergency department, clinical laboratory, pharmacy, etc.) and digitize the information in some common clinical coding format. Then one needs to encrypt it (thanks to an act of Congress, HIPAA, which will be discussed later). Finally, one has to move the information out onto the Internet and send it somewhere to be decoded and used. In other words, you have to do exactly the same things you need to do to make an enterprise system function properly.

If managing information networks was so easy to do, why did only 20 percent of U.S. hospitals have a functioning intranet, that is, a high-speed internal communications network, as late as 1998?[10] Intranets were a 1970s technology for networking computers at high speed inside an enterprise, invented at Xerox's famous Palo Alto Research Center. The answer to this question is simple: information systems linking departments had a far lower funding priority than the latest and slickest version of a laboratory information system or a new billing system.

As we will see in Chapter 5, the Internet has become a vehicle by which power over healthcare knowledge and decision making is shifting to consumers. The real leverage for hospitals in using the Internet comes from assisting in that shift toward consumers. Hospital executives will come to view Internet applications as a rich and diverse toolbox for restructuring their relationships with consumers and reducing the cost of resolving their health problems. Equally important, the Internet will support business process outsourcing, replacing many inadequately performing in-house administrative and (some) clinical processes with electronic processes managed by others, which are less costly and more responsive and transparent to their users.

Improving Service to Consumers

Many hospitals enrage consumers with awkward and user-unfriendly scheduling and chronically inept and unresponsive billing systems. The only way to make an appointment or check the status of a bill is to telephone the scheduling or billing office and endure an often lengthy wait on hold. Fixing these problems through network computing is a major opportunity for hospitals to use the Internet, but to do this, these processes need to be digitized in order to be accessible through electronic networks.

Scheduling, billing, medical information management, prescribing and renewing prescriptions, patient education, and dozens more processes need to be renovated electronically to make them accessible to consumers from outside the organization. There is no technical reason why patients cannot check the status of their bills over the Internet or make appointments or retrieve test results. Making this ability available will require patience, leadership from hospital boards and senior management, funding, and most important, a partnership between the IT vendors, the hospital's IT staff, and the departmental managers whose processes must be redesigned so that the consumer can connect to them from home.

Personal Health Records

Internet connectivity also makes it possible for hospitals, working with their physicians, local pharmacies, and other health providers to create personal health records (PHRs) that the consumers own and direct. At the consumer's discretion, this record can be sent to any facility where a family member receives care and can also be used at home to review medical histories and problems. The most obvious application will be replacing the shoeboxes in which many mothers store their children's immunization and other important health records with a convenient and easily accessible electronic record maintained on a hospital or health system server.

This record can also be "backed up" onto a so-called "smart card," a plastic card with a computer chip, or tiny "mass storage devices" connected to universal serial bus (USB) ports, which consumers can carry with them if they leave the community. Hospitals or doctors in other communities can then read the enclosed data if the consumer needs healthcare away from home. (This will require developing standard coding schemes that permit smart cards or storage devices to be read by different computer systems.)

A number of Internet start-up companies attempted to supply consumers with PHRs (including Dr.Koop.com) with less than dazzling results. Self-reported PHRs are likely to contain significant gaps in patient history and may not be sufficiently accurate or detailed to be clinically useful. The fact that self-reported records do not link to hospital or physician records means that they will contain only those things consumers themselves remember.

This makes hospitals potentially critical actors in creating PHRs for consumers. Hospitals can organize their computing networks to create PHRs for their patients, populating the PHR with information from the hospital's records. While health plans may have a similar capability (e.g., populating the PHR from their claims information), they will be handicapped by the fact that patient records were created for billing, not care management purposes. In addition, consumer concern that employers may gain access to their PHR, and thus to a comprehensive file of their confidential health information, will further handicap health plans as suppliers of consumer PHRs.

To supply a secure personal health record, hospitals would have to digitize patient information into an electronic medical record (discussed in Chapter 2) and then abstract the subset of information needed for a functioning PHR and store it in a secure "box" on a hospital or outside vendor server. Consumers would also have to authorize their physicians, local pharmacies, and other health services locations to contribute a consumer's medical encounter information (diagnoses, test results, prescriptions, etc.) to be uploaded into the hospital-assisted PHR.

An important test of this strategy is being pursued by the Cerner Corporation in the community of Winona, Minnesota, which has ubiquitous fiberoptic broadband in every home and provider site. In this community, the local hospital is collaborating with Cerner to provide all citizens with a web-based tool on their computer desktop for communicating with and managing their relationship to the hospital and the rest of the care system. This desktop tool will eventually contain a PHR. This system is expected to be live and operating by mid-2003.[11]

Outsourcing

The ability for hospitals to use the Internet to move clinical and administrative information into and out of the organization opens up the possibility that hospitals may be able to outsource—that is, to contract with outside firms—for many of the business functions they have struggled to perform effectively with their own hospital administrative staff.

Hospitals have traditionally been willing to outsource their "hotel management" functions—food service (to, e.g., Sodexho-Marriott), housekeeping (to, e.g., Servicemaster), laundry, and so forth (Figure 3.1). These decisions were easy to justify because they resulted in increased cost efficiency. Also, these were not controver-

Figure 3.1: Hospital Departments Outsourced

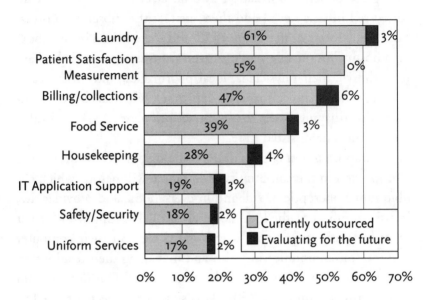

Source: Burmahl, B. 2001. "Percent of Hospitals Outsourcing Business/Support Functions." *Health Facilities Management.* [Online information, retrieved 12/20/02.] http:www.hospitalconnect.com/jsp/article.jsp?dcrpath=AHA/ NewsStory_Article/data/HFMMAGAZINE67&domain=HFMMAGAZINE.

sial decisions because the functions outsourced were not perceived to be central to the hospital's mission.

However, the Internet will make it possible to expand the list of outsourced services to the full suite of core business applications, including information processing and technology management, billing and collections, human resource management, and materials management. As a matter of fact, hospital outsourcing budgets for IT alone grew by 14 percent in 2002 and will grow more than 19 percent in 2003.[12] These functions are also not the core business of the hospital—patient care is the core business. Nevertheless, they are crucial to effective operations, and the failure to perform them reliably exposes the institution to market and financial risk.

THE COMING REVOLUTION IN HEALTH SOFTWARE

What makes outsourcing hospital functions increasingly practical is a revolution in how software is maintained and managed. Administrative and clinical software will reside not, as it does today, in the hundreds of computers at the desks of hospital personnel. Rather, complex clinical and administrative software will be "hosted" on powerful servers in a vendor's data center remote from the hospital. Hospital personnel will tie into these servers on high-bandwidth Internet connections through the web browser on their own computers. The heavy lifting—the data processing and system maintenance—will be handled in the vendor's data center at a location outside the community through application service provider (ASP) technology.

The complexity and, more importantly, the cost of maintaining, updating, and troubleshooting software applications will be markedly reduced by centralizing them in a single data center. It will not be necessary to change the code in everyone's computer in the hospital, as is done today, to upgrade or improve a computing application. Responsibility for keeping the system operating smoothly and continuously is the vendor's, not the hospital's.

The complexity of both clinical and financial IT for hospitals will come "out of the wall" in the hospital room, the operating suite, or the outpatient clinic. In IT jargon, this is called "thin client" architecture, meaning that one does not need high-performance computing at the user's end of the health system. The intelligence will be in the network the hospital (or physician or other user) taps into.

This will be particularly helpful for smaller hospitals that could not afford advanced computer applications under the old model. They will pay for sophisticated computer applications, like the clinical navigational system described in Chapter 2, on a subscription basis depending on how much they use the services. They will not need their own IT specialists in the hospital.

Application service providers will also make it possible for large or small hospitals to share administrative support with smaller hospitals or physician groups on an as-needed basis. There has been a shared-services tradition in hospitals for the past 30 years; the Internet will dramatically expand the capacity to share services and help hospitals large and small reduce their clerical and administrative staffing to concentrate their scarce resources on the clinical services that patients see and use.

Consumers will probably not notice any tangible difference between health services supported from inside the hospital and those supported by remote computing, except that the systems will be faster and waste less of their time in registration, billing, and other consumer-facing functions. However, hospitals will save money using these services that can be used to retain their nursing staffs and provide better customer service.

It Won't Happen Overnight

The emergence of these outsourcing capabilities will not happen overnight. ASP is off to a slow and sputtering start in healthcare. Fierce competition will take place between IT service firms—large consulting firms like First Consulting Group, Computer Sciences Corporation, Cap Gemini Ernst & Young, and Accenture; IT outsourcing vendors like Electronic Data Systems and Perot Systems; and IT product vendors like General Electric (GE), IBM, and Siemens, who have integrated from hardware into software and services—as well as hospital systems themselves that have special or unique service offerings.

This phenomenon of outsourced hospital administrative and clinical services can be expected to emerge, not over a few months, but over the next ten years, driven by the successful execution of remote computing models. In a decade, business process outsourcing may be a $100 billion business in healthcare. It will be characterized by significant price competition among IT vendors. The trend will also will be accelerated by the periodic cash flow and capital funding crises that hospitals experience. As it becomes more difficult for hospitals to borrow money, management will turn to "renting" or subscribing to business and clinical IT as an alternative to capital spending for IT.

As with any change in hospital operations, fierce cultural resistance to shared administrative and clinical services can be expected from hospital department heads and the physicians they support. A bold attempt in the late 1990s by a large Catholic hospital chain, Catholic Healthcare West, to "virtualize" administrative and support services across their system was a colossal multi-hundred-million-dollar failure. This failure was due to poor execution and fierce resistance from local and regional hospital bureaucracies.

Nevertheless, a more agile, responsive, and networked hospital system seems an inevitable, if painful, adaptation to an era of constrained public and private healthcare payment. Steven Goldman of Lehigh University has written extensively on this networked management model, which he has termed "agility."[13] This movement was directly responsible for the renaissance in manufacturing in the United States during the 1980s and early 1990s, as well as in the success of newer technology firms such as Cisco and Dell that were built around networked, collaborative, high-performance IT.

It was *not* a voluntary process. Many of the newer firms simply did not have the time to construct completely integrated manufacturing and marketing functions. Competitive exigencies forced them to craft electronic networks of suppliers and distributors to bring their technologies to market. Many of the older firms that made this adaptation in automobile manufacture, steel fabrication, and so on, did so because they faced ruin from overseas competition and pressure from their customers for higher product quality and more responsive customer service.

It is a troublesome reality that hospitalization exposes patients to risks that have nothing to do with their reason for being admitted in the first place. These risks include the risk of hospital-borne infections, adverse drug reactions, anesthesia problems, and other potential preventable threats to patient safety. Hospital executives have been uncertain of how to respond to reports of the prevalence of patient safety problems. Automating clinical processes is still very expensive, and hospital executives continue to question how significant an economic return these technologies will generate. Creating a safe, customer-friendly hospital experience that does not burn out caregivers with unnecessary clerical tasks will require a significant IT investment. The benefit-to-cost ratio of hospital IT will improve in future years as these technologies mature and become easier to use.

Will it be worth the price paid? Only if board and management leadership are intolerant of the excuses for delivering a substandard product to the communities they serve. Chapter 8 discusses how to anticipate the problems of transforming clinical and management cultures and how hospital managers, boards, and medical staffs can approach this challenge with their eyes open.

NOTES

1. Stevens, R. 1989. *In Sickness and in Wealth: American Hospitals in the 20th Century.* Baltimore, MD: Johns Hopkins University Press.

2. Goldsmith, J. 1981. *Can Hospitals Survive? The New Competitive Healthcare Market.* Chicago: Dow-Jones Irwin. Levit, K., C. Smith, C. Cowan, H. Lazenby, A. Sensenig, and A. Catlin. 2003. "Trends in U.S. Health Care Spending." *Health Affairs* 22 (1): 154–72.

3. Dorenfest, S. 2000. "The Decade of the 90s." *Healthcare Informatics* 17 (8): 64–67.

4. Goldsmith, J. C. 2002. "The Capital Conundrum: Balancing Needs Under Pressure." *Trustee* 55 (9): 10–13, 1.

5. Kane, C. K. 2001. "Physician Marketplace Report." [Online article; retrieved 12/6/02.] Chicago: American Medical Association. http://www.ama-assn.org /ama/upload/mm/363/practice200102.pdf.

6. Taylor, H., and R. Leitman, eds. 2001. "U.S. Trails Other English Speaking Countries in the Use of Electronic Medical Records and Electronic Prescribing." *Harris Interactive* 1 (28): 1–3.

7. Kleinke, J. D. 1998. "Release 0.0: Information Technology in the Real World." *Health Affairs* 17 (6): 23–37.

8. Institute of Medicine. 2000. *To Err Is Human: Building a Safer Health System.* Washington, DC: National Academy Press.

9. McDonald, C. J., J. M. Overhage, P. R. Dexter, L. Blevins, J. Meeks-Johnson, J. G. Suico, M. C. Tucker, and G. Schadowl. 1988. "Canopy Computing: Using the Web in Clinical Practice." *The Journal of the American Medical Association* 280 (15): 1325–28.

10. Deloitte Consulting. 1999. "Internet Health Strategy." Report. New York: Deloitte Consulting.

11. Cerner. 2000. "Winona Health Online, Cerner IQHealth's Pilot Community-based E-health Initiative, Is Live in Midwest City." [Online press release; retrieved 12/20/02.] Kansas City, MO: Cerner. http://www .cerner.com/aboutcerner/pressreleases.asp?id=994.

12. *Health Data Management.* 2002. "Survey: I.T. Major Source of Hospital Outsourcing." [Online information; retrieved 12/20/02]. http://www .healthdatamanagement.com/HDMSearchResultsDetails.cfm?DID=10382.

13. Goldman, S., and C. Graham, eds. 1999. *Agility in Healthcare: Strategies for Mastering Turbulent Markets.* San Francisco: Jossey-Bass.

CHAPTER 4

Physicians

PHYSICIANS ARE THE United States' most privileged and respected professional group. Despite the slings and arrows of managed care, physicians are also among the wealthiest professionals in
the United States. Wealth and power, however, have not brought
physicians the peace or sense of satisfaction one would have hoped.
Published reports on physician practices suggest that significant
numbers of physicians plan to retire in their 50s, well short of a
full professional career.[1] If these reports prove accurate, the United
States could face a serious shortage of practicing physicians as the
nation's 76 million baby boomers begin experiencing serious chronic
illness in the coming decades.

Sadly, given how important their work is, physicians function
in an environment of barely contained chaos. At least a part of the
problem is logistical. Most physicians practice in two places: the
hospital (whose troubled information systems were discussed in
the previous chapter) and their offices. In the vast majority of cases,
there is no functioning information link between these two sites.

Moreover, physicians' offices are awash in paper—patient records, prescriptions, medical journals, faxes, and telephone messages.
Technically sophisticated in their personal and professional lives,

physicians have nonetheless lagged in adopting modern information technology to support their practices.

THE PHYSICIAN AWAKENS AS GULLIVER

During the late 1980s, the unwritten and highly favorable social contract between physicians and society began undergoing revision. The pressures of rising health costs, particularly on private employers, encouraged an increased adoption of managed care. Narrowly construed, managed care involved establishing contractual relationships between physicians, hospitals, and other providers and health plans that limited the cost of care to predefined rates.

However, more broadly, these contracts gave health insurers the power to review and modify physicians' treatment plans to ensure that they were medically appropriate (with the goal of minimizing the cost).

The advent of managed care contracts massively complicated the business operations of most medical practices. They not only reduced physician fees but also increased their expenses. Because there are hundreds of health insurance plans with different coverage, review criteria, rates, and administrative procedures, health providers of all stripes found themselves bound like Gulliver by an emerging bureaucratic enterprise whose fundamental economic purpose was hostile to their own.

The practical reality of these changes was that physicians could not count on being paid for medical care that cost more than a few hundred dollars without obtaining prior approval from a health plan. Physicians were forced to double or triple their office staffs, in some cases, to manage all these new transactions, which depended largely on telephone calls, fax transmittals, and written correspondence. The increasingly complex logistics of medical practice claimed an increasing percentage of the physicians' workday, subtracting from time available for patients and family.

THE HIDDEN TOLL

No one appreciates having his or her income reduced. No one likes having his or her professional judgment or moral commitment questioned. It is not difficult to understand why the diminution of professional autonomy, incomes, and moral authority that physicians have experienced in the past decade would be unpleasant and stressful to them. But the increasing logistical complexity of physician practice has also taken a hidden toll on physicians. It has interfered with their intellectual development and ability to continue growing as professionals.

Physicians are intellectually curious, investigative, and empirical. They were the children who took things apart to see how they worked (and often succeeded in putting them back together). Many physicians were fascinated by the scientific portion of their medical training and continue to think of themselves, at least in part, as scientists. As the years in practice mount up and medical practice becomes more routine and repetitive, physicians yearn for new knowledge and ideas. The fact that they find gratifying this yearning increasingly difficult may be as important a contributor to professional burnout as the stress.

As the logistical complexity of professional practice has grown and administrative and familial obligations have grown alongside them, many physicians have found it difficult, if not impossible, to keep up with the exciting scientific discoveries taking place not only in their own disciplines but also in the underlying biological science as well.

Physicians see tantalizing glimpses of this progress in newspapers and the business and professional press. Unfortunately, however, a monthly hospital-sponsored continuing medical education session and interaction with drug detail persons may be the most important sources of new knowledge for the typical practicing physician. The channels through which knowledge passes to practicing physicians are narrow, convoluted, and inefficient.

ARE PROFESSIONALS INHERENTLY RESISTANT TO ADOPTING NEW TECHNOLOGY?

Physicians have sometimes been blamed for slowing the spread of computerization in healthcare. Some observers have speculated that physicians are technophobic and have resisted adopting modern IT because they feel it erodes their professional autonomy.

Physician attitudes toward technology may be described as mildly Luddite. Alissa Spielberg writes about the physician reaction to the telephone, a technology that unquestionably transformed medical practice:

> From its inception, the telephone engendered [physician] concerns about privacy and security. Its intrusiveness into daily living and personal space made the telephone particularly vexing to early users who complained about solicitations, eavesdroppers, and even "wire transmitted germs" . . . As the telephone became embedded within American culture, patients expected their physicians to be accessible at any time for almost any reason. Physicians felt vulnerable, even "slaves," to a potential barrage of calls from anxious patients.[2]

Nevertheless, Spielberg observes, physicians felt morally obligated to be available over the telephone and eventually embraced the new technology.

> Although patients and physicians recognized potential problems with confidentiality and care over the telephone, most also conceded that the telephone had dramatically altered the patient-physician relationship by making private what was once public.[3]

To characterize physicians as technophobic is innacurate. In my sample of several thousand physician contacts and friends, most are fascinated with technology. They adopt it aggressively in their own fields of specialization and are constantly scanning the horizon for new technology that may help them in their work (Figure 4.1). They buy technologically advanced automobiles, home computers, and sound equipment and gravitate to "gear-intensive" sports like sailing and skiing.

For the generation of physicians now entering practice, using computers is as natural as breathing. However, those who came to computers in midlife have experienced great frustration in mastering the complexity of allegedly intuitive computer operating systems. They perform some function, push "enter," and nothing happens, or the wrong thing happens. The computer-use experience is the antithesis of the surgeon's commanding the operating suite: putting out one's hand and having a scalpel magically appear in one's palm. Computers simply do not work this way.

The medical education process has materially contributed to physicians' disability in learning about computers. Although they remain intellectually curious, the irreverence and spontaneity many young people bring to medical education is, sadly, extinguished by a combination of exhaustion and the stern disapproval of their teachers.

By the time they enter practice, physicians are already over-stressed, time-famished, and fault-intolerant. If something does not work right the first time or takes too long to produce results, physicians have developed reflexes that cause them to move on rather than to tinker until they get the result they want. Ironically, younger physicians are actually harder to please with computer applications, because they have higher expectations of ease of use and functionality than their older colleagues, who still mistrust their reflexes and command of the technology.

Having said all this, physicians across the board have begun using computers in their personal lives. More than 90 percent of them are online, a markedly higher percentage than among the broad consumer population, although only 56 percent can access the Internet from their offices.[4] If they have not mastered taking down MP3 audio files or instant messaging like their kids, they have conquered e-mail, and many manage their investments online.

Physicians have become moderately sophisticated users of modern network computing.

INFORMATION TECHNOLOGY AND MEDICAL PRACTICE

Applying IT to their practices, however, has been a different story. Most physicians still practice in overtaxed small businesses. Because every dollar of practice expense is viewed as income forgone, physicians (even in large group practices) typically starve their businesses for capital, of which computer technology is part. Over time, physicians evolved manual clinical and financial systems that work for them, but at a price: increasingly costly clerical support to manage the flow of patient information, scheduling, and, particularly, billing and interaction with health insurers.

Replacing these manual systems with computerized systems, furthermore, is time consuming and painful. For group practice managers, one sure way to get fired is to bungle the installation of a computer system and impede the flow of funds to physicians.

In fairness to doctors, however, there have also been problems with the "product." Historically, computer systems for physicians (as well as hospitals) have been difficult and expensive to install and use. All too often, business software for medicine has been riddled with bugs and is difficult to connect to other programs or systems on which the software depends.[5] Vendors of medical software have often misrepresented the capabilities of their products and have had difficulty in delivering the improvements in care and cash flow they promised.

As a consequence, physicians and managers have become appropriately skeptical about whether new systems can help them and have delayed making what they perceive as risky new investments in IT. Physicians have a high functional "hurdle" that information systems must surmount for them to be readily accepted and used.

Figure 4.1: Internet, Web Site, and E-mail Usage by Physicians

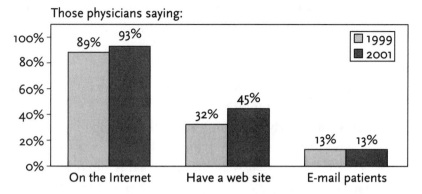

Source: "Strategic Health Perspectives, 1997–1999." *Computing in the Physician's Practice,* 2001.

Specifically, they must make practicing medicine demonstrably easier and more financially rewarding.

PHYSICIANS' ADOPTION OF IT IN OTHER COUNTRIES

American physicians lag considerably behind physicians in other countries in taking up and using computer technology in their medical practices. According to a recent Harris Interactive study, only 17 percent of primary care physicians and 12 percent of specialists in the United States reported using electronic medical records in 2000. On the primary care side, this compares to 52 percent in New Zealand and 59 percent in the United Kingdom. On the specialty side, utilization is lower: 14 percent of New Zealand specialists and 22 percent of specialists in the United Kingdom (many of whom are salaried employees of Britain's National Health Service) report using electronic medical records.[6]

U.S. physicians also lag behind their colleagues in the United Kingdom in using electronic prescribing of drugs. Only 9 percent of U.S. primary care physicians and 6 percent of specialists reported using some form of electronic prescribing in 2000. In New Zealand, by contrast, 52 percent of primary care physicians and 14 percent of specialists reported prescribing drugs electronically. In Britain, 87 percent of primary care physicians and 16 percent of specialists reported electronic prescribing.[7]

What is particularly interesting about these comparisons is that there is almost no primary care group practice in these two countries. GPs are almost exclusively solo and partnership practitioners and practice outside the control of hospitals. Hospital-dependent specialists lag considerably behind their freestanding GP colleagues in adopting computer technology to aid their practices.

THE BENEFITS FOR PHYSICIANS

Information technology will soon transform medical practice. It will markedly ease the difficulties in communication not only between doctors and patients, but also among physicians. Although it may take a decade or more, IT will eventually conquer the tangle of paper transactions at the heart of our healthcare payment system, making the patient's part of this transaction as simple as swiping a credit card to purchase a shirt.

Most importantly, however, IT will assist materially in helping keep physicians' minds alive and in closing the gap between the front lines of medical practice and the research laboratories and seats of technical innovation in medicine where new knowledge and tools are created.

A major barrier to adoption of modern business software for physician practices was that it required physicians to make a significant capital expenditure. Incurring debt of any kind often required physicians to guarantee the debt personally, heaping business debt on top of large mortgages, automobile leases, medical school loans, and who knows what else. Also, recall that the software was of questionable reliability. Principally for this reason, only 17 percent of physicians' office medical records are electronic, as of this writing.[8]

For many years, hospitals and health insurers have used remote computing applications, where data processing was managed by an outside firm, and data were moved to and from the outside firm through modems and dedicated, high-bandwidth telephone connections like T1 lines. Electronic commerce in healthcare did not begin with the Internet. Indeed, it has been conducted for 25 years. Electronic commerce through dedicated lines was the backbone of such large IT vendors as Shared Medical Systems and Electronic Data Systems.

Most physicians were locked out of electronic commerce in medicine because of the small scale of their computing needs and the high cost of the dedicated T1 telephone connection (which could range from $1,000 to $5,000 a month). With the Internet and increasingly affordable high-bandwidth services such as ISDN and now DSL and cable, even small physician practices can afford to connect to remote computing vendors for one-tenth as much money.

The firms that physicians can connect to can not only process their medical claims for them but can also support electronic patient records and patient e-mail access to their physicians.[9] Instead of incurring a $50,000 to $250,000 capital expense and worrying about whether their office staff could install the software, physicians can now dial up business and clinical systems through a web browser and pay a modest subscription fee.

The technology used here, as discussed earlier, is an application service provider (ASP). Under ASP, complex software is not maintained in the physicians' office on expensive, high-end servers. Rather, the software comes "out of the wall." It is accessed through a web browser and fast Internet connection and is maintained centrally by the vendor in a data center at some remote location.

All the office-based physician needs is a modestly powered desktop computer, training for the office staff, and the patience to reconfigure his or her current billing and record-keeping systems.

Physicians can now purchase computer support for their practices that once only large group practices and hospitals could afford. As of this writing, ASP is still a developing business in the physician world, but the scale economies and modest costs are a great boon to physicians who view every capital or operating expense as a deduction from their monthly payroll check.

Eventually, this office-based software will be connected electronically to the health plans, which will accept, evaluate, and pay physician claims electronically, without the physician's office needing to generate paper bills. Reducing the need to handle paper medical claims will also markedly reduce the administrative costs of health plans. The patients' portion of the bill will be predetermined, based on their unique health insurance coverage (which is part of each patient's computer file). The patients' share will then be billed to their credit card at the time of service, reducing both accounts receivable and the physician's office clerical costs.

Again, although it may take up to a decade, eventually most physicians' offices will free themselves from paper records and billing systems. When they make the conversion from paper record and bills to digital systems, physicians will be able to reduce their clerical employment by as much as one-half and rededicate their nursing personnel to clinical, rather than office, tasks.

Consumers will experience all of this as much easier and more hassle-free service from their physicians' office. They will not be asked to re-register every time they see their physicians because their computer file will "remember" all the pertinent insurance information from the last visit. Rather, consumers will be able to make appointments and register for their visits from home via their web browser.

HOW WILL PHYSICIANS USE NETWORK COMPUTING?

Although physicians have taken to the Internet in large numbers in their personal lives, they have been thus far profoundly reluctant to incorporate Internet applications into their practices. While physicians are beginning to use e-mail to network with professional colleagues, estimates as of December 2002 suggest only 23 percent use e-mail to communicate with their patients.[10] Group Health Cooperative of Puget Sound (Wash.) has seen a significant increase, with 60 percent of e-mails replacing phone calls and 20 percent replacing an office visit, freeing up physicians for other things.[11]

Although physicians have been barraged with opportunities to participate in online medical communities and gain access to medical information through web portals, the depth and breadth of physician participation has been surprisingly modest. Only 16 percent of physicians who see patients 65 or more hours a week reported that they use e-mail and online consultations.[12] From the patient's perspective, there is substantial unrequited interest in e-mail linkage to their doctors. According to a CyberDialog survey in 1999, 48 percent of patients want e-mail links to their doctors.[13]

Some physicians have argued that their reluctance to open an e-mail channel of communication to patients stems from the lack of payment by health insurers. What they may not consider is that the same lack of payment applies to the time consuming and frustrating game of telephone tag physicians presently play with their patients. The critical difference is that telephone contacts are filtered through office staff, whereas physicians receive e-mail communication directly. Clinical spam and "cyberchondria" have frozen many doctors' willingness to open the e-mail channel to patients.

IMPROVING PHYSICIAN-PATIENT COMMUNICATION

E-mail Communications

Physician-patient communication via e-mail is a complex issue, and the leisurely pace of adoption of this communications tool is understandable. The Health Insurance Portability and Accountability

Act of 1996 (HIPAA) requires that physician-patient communication containing personally identifiable medical information be encrypted and access be restricted to protect patient privacy. While the technical issues surrounding these requirements are not complex, they do represent at least a temporary restraint to free flow of communication.

Nonetheless, once privacy and security issues have been surmounted, e-mail has demonstrable advantages over telephone communication for sustaining the doctor-patient relationship. E-mail can be triaged by office staff, and routine requests like prescription renewals that do not require the physician's direct intervention can be managed without disturbing him or her.

Moreover, the subset of e-mail communications that require a physician response can be managed "asynchronously," that is, when physicians have time to read and respond. The fact that time and content of communication "threads" with patients can be printed out or copied into the patient's electronic medical record makes these safer forms of communication than telephone calls from a medical-legal standpoint.

However, the potential for Internet-supported physician-patient communication extends far beyond the exchange of e-mail. Unlike the telephone, e-mail can support a tremendous density and richness of content. Rather than being passive recipients of Internet-generated scientific information and news articles from patients (as most are today), physicians will begin archiving information on diseases and medical conditions they see frequently and attaching these articles to patient communications as "homework."

Rather than repeating the same information orally to patient after patient, physicians can give their patients what John Glaser, chief information officer at Partners Healthcare System in Boston, has called an "information prescription" after diagnosis to guide the patient's education and self-care. This information can be as rich and dense as patient preference dictates, from journal articles rich with citations and hypertext links to content sites to simple step-by-step guidelines for self-evaluation and management.

Procedure-oriented physicians can convey information to patients both pre- and post-procedure to ensure that patients are adequately prepared and equipped to manage their own end of the "transaction" (diet, medication, clinical support requirements, etc.). Comprehensive e-mail communication can strengthen the patient's and family's ability to manage medical problems and make use of the limited time with the physician more efficient.

Disease Management

Powerful Internet-based applications can maintain more or less continuous contact between physicians and patients with unstable conditions. Physicians will be able to offer disease-management software accessible through the Internet to track the patient's condition and guide the patient's and family's response to the disease risk. Managing conditions like asthma, diabetes, hypertension, and some forms of cancer require not only adherence to dietary and pharmaceutical guidelines, but continuous monitoring of the patient's condition. These conditions are ideal for online disease management, as the computer software will perform many of the surveillance functions that otherwise would have required patients to be hospitalized.

Monitoring can be structured according to clinical guidelines that measure the desirable patient vital signs and automatically report variances to a monitoring station, alerting physicians or nurses to potential health problems in the home before they become serious enough to require an emergency room visit or a hospital admission. These guidelines can be "projected" from the intelligent clinical management systems (the advanced electronic medical records systems discussed Chapter 3) in the home, hospital, or physician clinic in which the physician works.

Rather than relying principally on direct contact through physician visits, much of this monitoring and evaluation will be supported from home by medical software that patients can access through a web page maintained by the physician or by outside vendors or their hospital system. Thus, the physician's protection and advice can be extended and strengthened by disease-management software that reaches into the patient's home around the clock (24/7).

Second Opinions and Other Consultations

Internet connectivity through broadband will dramatically increase the ease with which medical consultation can take place throughout the world. Prior to the availability and extensive use of Internet, requests from physicians for specialty consultation were generated by telephone and were followed by paper medical records, x-rays, lab reports, and other information for consultation to take place. Sometimes these records are hand carried by the patient to a scheduled appointment.

With broadband Internet connections, it will be possible for complex patient records, including the medical record itself, digital radiological images, pathology reports, and even voice files to be sent instantaneously anywhere in the world as attachments to e-mail. Partners Health System (the Massachusetts General/Brigham and Women's Hospitals in Boston) has allied itself with Duke University Medical Center, Johns Hopkins University, and The Cleveland Clinic Foundation to create a consortium to provide international electronic second-opinion consultations. Their consortium is called WorldCare. [14,15]

This ability will make it possible for physicians to seek advice from colleagues anywhere in the world about one's medical condition without one having to physically travel. Although the Internet is completely oblivious to geographic and political boundaries, complex licensure issues will be problematic until telemedicine legislation is modified.

It is still not clear at this writing, beyond teleradiology, how big an economic opportunity Internet-assisted telemedicine can become. At least for the foreseeable future, most of the economic opportunities for healthcare organizations will continue to be generated by patient visits. Thus, information exchange, even consultation on the specifics of a patient's problem, may be an important prelude to, but not a substitute for, the visit, during which something is actually done to resolve the patient's problem.

PEER CONTACT

Although physicians learn an increasing amount about their disciplines from interaction with the cyber-assisted patient, contact with their professional peers and colleagues is still the principal mechanism for transmitting new medical knowledge. Physicians tend to be highly gregarious within their disciplines (e.g., internal medicine, orthopedics, radiology).

Specialty societies have realized that they are trusted sources of medical knowledge and can leverage their prestige and legitimacy as representatives of their disciplines to create clinical content. These organizations, such as the American College of Cardiology and the American Academy of Orthopedic Surgeons, were traditionally reluctant to foster consensus about best clinical practices for their members because of concerns about antitrust or competitive relationships within or between disciplines (e.g., who is better qualified to perform back surgery—orthopedic surgeons or neurosurgeons?).

However, the ability to put the stamp of professional legitimacy on practice guidelines, based upon peer-reviewed research, puts these societies in the position of creating valuable content both for consumer and professional web sites, and for clinical operating systems like the intelligent electronic medical records discussed in the previous chapter.

Connectivity is making it easier for colleagues to convene in cyberspace, not only to consult on specific cases (as discussed above), but also to exchange ideas, collaborate in applying for grants, conduct research activity, and organize to influence funding decisions for research and for clinical care in Washington and state capitols. It is also enabling physicians to remain in contact with their chiefs and colleagues who trained them in medical school and residency training without having to travel.

Contact and learning across disciplines is more complex. This is the ultimate source of competitive advantage of multispecialty physician organizations like the Mayo Clinic and the Permanente Medical Groups of Kaiser. The culture of successful multispecialty groups fosters easy interaction between physicians of different specialties. This culture makes it possible for an internist to reach colleagues in psychiatry, neurology, or infectious disease easily with patient-related questions that relate to their disciplines. Electronic connectivity will multiply these interactions by making it unnecessary for both parties to be simultaneously connected or physically proximate.

Relying on a trusted professional colleague to filter knowledge and focus it on a specific clinical problem is far more efficient than conducting one's own literature search or sallying forth onto the Internet to find the answer. The best clinical care can be found in institutions where peer communication is easy and open.

It will be many years before the virtual version of this easy peer connection can be fostered in the medical part of the Internet, again in part due to medical-legal concerns. Medicine is so fragmented, and the knowledge base so diverse, that a workable peer-to-peer solution to locating and retrieving medical knowledge seems unlikely to appear any time soon. However, it is logical to expect that it will eventually happen.

In the meantime, the Internet will make it easier for physicians to communicate with each other and foster network relationships that extend beyond the walls of the specific institutions in which physicians practice. Groupware like Lotus Notes has long made it possible for clinical and research teams that are dispersed geographically to work on common projects. Physicians' natural curiosity and gregariousness seem likely to find new outlets in virtual collaboration on the Internet.

Physicians are likely to find that searching for and retaining new medical knowledge will be much easier in a decade than it is now. Already, since 1994, physicians have been able to gain access to the National Library of Medicine's MEDLINE Service through a web browser. Medical journals have raced to make their content available to physicians and other subscribers online. Portals and content aggregators such as WebMD and Medscape have contributed medical news reporting to online access to journals and health information databases to helping physicians remain current.

PDAS

The fundamental ethic of practicing physicians, that the bulk of their medical knowledge must be readily accessible in their memories or in text form, needs revisiting in light of new capabilities for searching for and archiving knowledge. A Charlottesville, Virginia–based company, Unbound Medicine, has developed a Palm-based knowledge management tool to help physicians scan the medical literature and store relevant new knowledge where they can find it easily and quickly, for example, on their personal digital assistant (PDA).

When physicians subscribe to their service, which is called CogniQ, they list all of the medical journals they follow. When new issues of these journals become available, the tables of contents and abstracts are loaded onto the physicians' PDA from the CogniQ server. Physicians can scan the new articles and choose those of interest to be archived in their box on the Unbound Medicine server, in abstract or full-text form. They can then be read at leisure.

As physicians move through their practice day, they can also enter questions into the PDA through its Graffiti function. When they synchronize their PDA to their personal computer, the PC will send the question or search item to the Unbound Medicine server, which will use a search tool to identify and store relevant articles that address the question in the physician's box on their server.

Thus, questions that would have been lost end up getting answered and stored in an easily retrievable fashion. Over time, the server retains the entire stream of answers to questions and relevant journal articles as a personalized "knowledge archive," making it unnecessary for the physician to retain the new knowledge in his or her memory. This service will evolve from being modem dependent to being wireless as it becomes more widely available. It is obvious that as the software improves, services like this will incorporate speech recognition that obviates the need for scribbling or tapping on the PDA's tiny screen.

Physicians like PDAs because they can slip them into the pockets of their lab coats. According to a recent Harris Interactive Poll, more than one-quarter of physicians owned PDAs by early 2001, although only about 18 percent use them for clinical purposes.[16] Significantly, however, this number doubled in just a year's time, suggesting a very rapid adoption curve. It is now rare to see a medical resident without a PDA.

Not only will the PDA contain knowledge management tools, but they will also carry pharmaceutical software that helps physicians select drugs, evaluate their risks and interactions, and prescribe from anywhere. PDAs also contain decision-support tools developed specifically for the physician's medical specialty, such as differential diagnosis programs. These programs will enable a physician to enter patient symptoms into the PDA and be led through a sequence of questions to a tentative diagnosis for the patient's problem. It is easy to envision the struggle for the PDA "desktop" (similar to the struggle for shelf space in the supermarket).

As it fuses with the cellular telephone, the PDA will evolve into an indispensable electronic extension of the physician that can link to his or her practice management software, electronic patient records, hospital laboratory and radiology departments, and to colleagues. Although it is taking longer than some observers expected, the PDA of 2005 will have storage and processing power comparable to today's laptop computers and integrate communications (wireless phone) and data-management functions.

As physicians realize this is technically possible, they will put tremendous pressure on vendors, their hospitals, and practice managers to make the required data linkages happen. As this occurs, physicians will be freed from the need to return telephone calls or to give verbal orders, enabling them to practice medicine "anytime, anywhere."

SURMOUNTING THE HOSPITAL-PHYSICIAN BARRIER

As Rosemary Stevens reminded us in *In Sickness and in Wealth,* tension has existed between hospitals and their physicians for most of the past century.[17] As managed care ramped up in the late 1980s and early 1990s, relationships between hospital management and physicians deteriorated. In many institutions, physician mistrust of hospital motivations and strategies is a dominant theme.

Mistrust

Although competitive tensions between physician-sponsored enterprises and hospitals have contributed to this problem, many physicians view the hospital as a battleship whose wake is sufficient to swamp the small boats it operates. The fact that hospitals and physicians have completely separate information domains complicates the ability to implement new clinical information systems.

The Hospital as Potential Information Source

Hospitals are presently committing major capital resources to computerize both operations and clinical services. As argued above, physician practices, even many large groups, are capital poor and thus lag in automating their processes and services. It is entirely possible given the present course that hospitals will complete this process a decade or more ahead of physicians, leaving what physicians "know" about their patients locked up in paper records and their memories.

When physicians do automate, if no compatibility standards are set in advance, they will use incompatible software and be unable to move clinical information between their systems and those of the hospital. This is obviously not optimal. Optimal patient care would require that the clinical team be able to access important clinical information about a patient at any place and at any time. Because hospitals have capital, and physicians, generally speaking, do not, hospitals could be a potential source for modern digital clinical information systems, as well as patient care support tools like disease management, for their physicians. If hospitals could help bring about a shared record format across their medical staffs, it would be easier for physicians to send patient information to one another for consultative purposes.

Historically, physicians have been extremely reluctant to permit hospitals access to their private practices. Many experiments by hospitals during the 1990s with salaried employment of physicians and with practice management support ended in costly failure. Physicians resisted installing inexpensive software that enabled them to perform remote order entry or retrieval of test results from hospitals because they thought it opened a portal that enabled hospital executives to understand their practice's economics.

Legal and Regulatory Barriers

Besides the mistrust discussed above, legal and regulatory barriers make linking hospitals and physicians difficult. Federal Medicare regulations forbid hospitals from offering physicians anything of value (including software and services) if it would influence their patterns of hospital utilization. These statutes were intended to prevent hospitals from, in effect, bribing physicians to bring their patients in. If compatible clinical software made it easier for physicians with a choice to use the facility that provided them the software, it might trigger fraud and abuse investigations.

Tax laws provide another barrier to the sharing of clinical software between hospitals and physicians. The Internal Revenue Code and state laws forbid not-for-profit hospitals (recall that 85 percent of all community hospitals are not-for-profit) from giving physicians (or anyone else) anything of value. The technical term for these gifts is "inurement of benefit." Free software or free installation of the software could be construed as inurement of benefit and thus could threaten a hospital's tax-exempt status.[18]

Given the overriding societal interest in encouraging a rapid movement to digital patient care systems, these laws should be amended to exempt clinical IT. Competitive advantage for specific providers could be eliminated by regulation that requires clinical information systems developed by different vendors to interoperate (that is, to use common record formats, coding conventions, messaging standards, etc.). This would mean that, once installed, physicians could use their clinical software in conjunction with any of the available local hospitals or retrieve information about their patients from any of them.

The fact that software and services could be provided on a dial-in basis without significant capital expenditures by hospitals on the physicians' behalf could help change some of the equation as well. The most expensive part of a physician office's digital conversion is transferring all of its existing patient records to digital form so they can be used by the information system. If these costs can be surmounted and physicians can obtain password-protected access to computerized patient records and clinical decision support from their offices, it would be a major boost to overall computerization.

Hospitals and Physicians Digitizing Patient Records Together

Ideally, hospitals and physicians should move together to digitize patient records. Technical opportunities exist for hospitals to create virtual private networks that segregate the physician's clinical records from those of the hospital (as well as the rest of the Internet), protect the physician's business autonomy and privacy, and still provide the transparency of information flow that is needed for optimal patient care. To do this will require physician leadership and "followership," whereby physicians place trust in their leaders to negotiate and represent their interests with hospital management on IT policy and priorities. Physicians have to be willing to wade into the battle over how digital medicine is organized and be assured that their concerns about autonomy and privacy are recognized.

HOW MUCH WILL PHYSICIANS REALLY AUTOMATE THEIR PRACTICES?

When you sum the potential impact of various information technologies across the physician's world, the aggregate impact is impressive. Information technology will *eventually* do the following:

1. Speed the flow of new knowledge to physicians and store it efficiently so physicians don't have to rely on their memories
2. Guide and assist in patient care itself, wherever the physician or patient may be at the moment
3. Free physicians from paper records and bills, reducing their practice expenses
4. Markedly improve and enrich communications with patients
5. Facilitate collaboration between physicians both in consultation and in learning

As with hospitals, this progress will not come easily, quickly, or cheaply. Moreover, not all physicians will be able to realize all of these benefits at the same time. Physicians practicing in larger groups and clinic settings will find these tools become available to them sooner simply because their organizations have the financial resources and personnel to make them happen and the capability of experimenting with these tools before adopting them wholesale. Physicians in private practice will have to overcome mistrust of their hospitals and each other and work with their colleagues to build data systems they can use from the office or from home.

However, what ails physicians stretches far beyond the curable logistical difficulties of medical practice itself. Information technology can make it far easier to practice medicine. In addition, if properly employed, IT can also make it more fun to practice medicine by enabling physicians to follow their curiosity and interests. What IT will be unable to do is to restore physicians' confidence in the importance and meaningfulness of what they are doing. At the root of medicine's midlife crisis is the nagging feeling on physicians' part that patients and society no longer trust them.

Consumers are sending physicians a message: be more available to us when we need your help, do not patronize us, and give us the information we need to help us manage our own health. The physicians who hear these messages develop new relationships with consumers and may find their practices acquire more meaning. It behooves healthcare executives to support physicians in this effort.

Physicians who grasp this capability effectively will also find that they can grow their practices and, by making more efficient use of their own time, still devote more time to the patients who need the personal contact. Information technology can extend the power of the physician's mind, a most valuable and fragile tool, and can help strengthen the doctor-patient relationship. As this relationship is improved, it may help lay the groundwork for a newer, more confident medicine.

Although they may not believe it, physicians retain extraordinary power in our health system. All too often, they have used that power to retard needed changes in health policy and management. With information technology, however, physicians have a marvelous opportunity to lead the transformation. Because they remain strategic actors, not only in health systems, but also in the lives of patients, physicians hold the key to "birthing" the digital transformation of the health system. By aggressively experimenting with IT and embracing its use by their colleagues and the health systems they animate, physicians can speed the adoption of these powerful new tools by a decade or more.

For further, in-depth readings on the benefits of digitization on physicians, I recommend *Digital Doctors* by Marshall de Graffenried Ruffin, Jr.[19]

NOTES

1. Silverman, J., and S. Peters. 2001. "Doctor Discontent." *Family Practice News* 31 (7): 33.

2. Spielberg, A. R. 1998. "On Call and Online: Sociohistorical, Legal, and Ethical Implications of E-mail for the Patient-Physician Relationship." *Journal of the American Medical Association* 280 (15): 1353–59.

3. Ibid.

4. Taylor, H., and R. Leitman. 2001. "New Data Show Internet, Website and Email Usage by Physicians All Increasing." *Harris Interative* 1 (8): 1–3.

5. Kleinke, J. D. 1998. "Release 0.0: Information Technology in the Real World." *Health Affairs* 17 (6): 23–27.

6. Taylor, H., and R. Leitman. 2001. "U.S. Trails Other English Speaking Countries in Use of Electronic Medical Records and Electronic Prescribing." *Harris Interactive* 1 (28): 1–3.

7. Ibid.

8. Ibid.

9. Monahan, T. 2001. "ASPs Offer Something That Healthcare Finds Increasingly Hard to Get." *Healthcare Informatics* 18 (2): 54, 56.

10. Stevens, L. 2002. "The Expansion of e-Health." *Medicine on the Net* 8 (12): 1–5.

11. Ibid.

12. Taylor, H., and R. Leitman. 2001. "The Increasing Impact of eHealth on Physician Behavior." *Harris Interactive* 1 (21): 1–9.

13. Cyber Dialogue. 1999. "Doctors are Missing Internet Health Opportunity." [Online information; retrieved 12/15/02.] http://www.cyberdialogue.com/news /releases/1999/10-12-cch-doctors.html.

14. Peiper, J. 2001. Partners HealthCare System. Personal communication, September.

15. Kowalcyzk, L. 2000. "Overseas Patients to Get 2nd Opinions Via Internet." *Boston Globe*, May 10.

16. Taylor, H., and R. Leitman. 2001. "Physicians' Use of Handheld Personal Computing Devices Increases From 15% in 1999 to 26% in 2001." *Harris Interactive* 1 (25): 1–4.

17. Stevens, R. 1989. *In Sickness and in Wealth: American Hospitals in the 20th Century*. Baltimore, MD: Johns Hopkins University Press.

18. Brauer, L. M., and C. F. Kaiser III. "Physician Incentive Compensation." [Online information; retrieved 1/2/02.] Washington, DC: Internal Revenue Service. http://www.irs.gov/pub/irs-tege/topicc00.pdf.

19. Ruffin, M. de Graffenried, Jr. 1999. *Digital Doctors*. Tampa, FL: American College of Physician Executives.

CHAPTER 5

The Consumer: Patient No More

USING THE HEALTH system is a quest for life-saving or life-changing knowledge. Measured against this end point, the contemporary health system in the United States has become increasingly user-unfriendly. The institutions of medical practice—hospitals, health plans, and physician organizations—have grown so large and become so intimidating that many of them dwarf those who give and receive care. As mechanisms for transmitting knowledge, healthcare organizations have become riddled with bureaucracy and institutional processes that impede the free flow of communication between patients and caregivers.

Moreover, as discussed in Chapter 1, healthcare institutions have become prisons of vital medical knowledge. The knowledge and wisdom that all the actors in healthcare seek from medical institutions is imprisoned in paper, in indecipherable notes and images, in journals and professional reports that are often written in a private language few can understand, and in the overtaxed memories of caregivers. New knowledge is flooding into the health system at an accelerating pace, but ensuring that this vital new knowledge actually reaches the practitioners and consumers who need it is an urgent piece of unfinished business.

93

Armed with unprecedented access to information by way of the Internet, consumers have begun to react angrily to this failure to deliver the solutions they think should be readily available. The health system is there to serve them, and through their taxes and forgone salaries, they pay most of its bills. Managing consumer expectations for compassionate and responsive advice and care is the central challenge facing our health system.

HOW TO TALK ABOUT THE "USER"

To begin this discussion, we need to confront directly the vocabulary problem. How we describe people in our health system is important and has significant consequences for how we think about them. In describing the role users play in the health system, traditional vocabulary and medical culture constrain us. The word "patient" increasingly fails to describe accurately the role of the user.

Healthcare professionals generally view with disdain the use of the term "consumer" or "customer" to describe the health system's "users" because they feel it commercializes the care relationship and demeans them as professionals. Physicians in particular resist commercial terminology, at least in part because they are uncomfortable with the economic implications of their professional power.

However, the traditional term that describes the health system's user as a "patient" (throughout this chapter, the term "patient" should be read with the current discussion in mind) is troublesome for several reasons. First, in many cases, it ignores the role of the family in the care process. The more profoundly ill or disabled the patient is, the more likely that the decision maker is the family or a key family member. Many forms of care, such as ambulatory surgery or cooperative care in rehabilitation, explicitly recognize the role of the family member as a participant in the care team. In the case of chronic care, a very significant majority of the care is actually rendered by a family member, not "official" health professionals.

Of course, people are not always in contact with the health system. At any given time, only a small fraction of the population, perhaps as few as 5 percent, are actually using the health system. When feeling well, they are not patients, and yet they play a role in the health system that the traditional vocabulary does not recognize. In the emerging genetic age, one may not have been officially diagnosed as "ill," yet one carries a complex and highly individual pattern of genetic risk. This person may not be a patient in the traditional sense, but is engaged, to some degree consciously, in managing that risk nonetheless.

Thus, although a person is not receiving care as a patient, he or she may be acquiring information about emerging health risks or medical problems that have not yet resulted in seeking care, arguing with the health insurer over paying a medical bill, participating in an online discussion of a medical issue, and so forth. When that step is taken, then, is that person a patient, or even a consumer, or merely a person living life?

Other problems arise with the term "patient." It connotes a passive role and suggests that this is a person with time to waste. One of my mentors in health services research, Dr. Odin Anderson, famously referred to the role of the patient in the traditional health system as that of the "breathing brick." This image in no way describes most users of the health system today. It is particularly inaccurate in describing the baby boom women who are, as discussed below, the "power users" in the present health system.

Consumers, on the other hand, make choices, and because they make choices, they exercise economic power. They weigh the value of the goods or services they are using and make decisions based on their value relative to alternative uses of their money. As consumers pay more of the healthcare bill out of their grocery money—a major trend in health insurance coverage in the future—this value-seeking behavior will play a larger role in their dialog with physicians.

WHO IS THE HEALTHCARE CONSUMER?

It is important to pause here and observe that the term "healthcare consumer" operationally refers to women. Women use significantly more health services than the men in their households. According to the National Center for Health Statistics, men have one-third fewer physician visits, outpatient visits, and hospital admissions than women.[1] More important, however, the woman in the household is likely to be the unofficial and unpaid general manager of her family's health.

Whether they are wives, daughters, sisters, aunts, or cousins, women typically control healthcare decisions not only for themselves, but also for multiple family members. According to *Our Bodies, Ourselves*, "women use the health system twice as often as men, not just for our own care but because we are so often responsible for children, partners, aging parents, and other relatives as well."[2] As a result, women control the distribution of almost two-thirds of all health spending.[3]

She is also more than likely the person who selects the health plan her family uses and the person responsible for seeing that the health plan pays her family's eligible medical expenses. She selects or influences the selection of the physician and hospitals that the family uses. She drives family members to and from the medical encounter. Finally, if an elderly, chronically ill person is in the household, she is the first line caregiver/care manager for that person.

THE TRADITIONAL KNOWLEDGE PATHWAY IN MEDICINE

Acquiring knowledge about our conditions and disease risk is the principal reason why people connect with the health system. The traditional framework for knowledge transmission in medicine, as depicted in Figure 5.1, has not changed materially since Hippocrates.

The consumer experiences some form of medical uncertainty.

Figure 5.1: Knowledge Transmission in Medicine, Twentieth Century

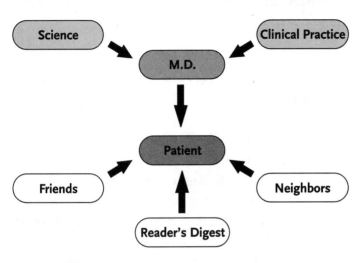

Source: Health Futures, Inc.

This uncertainty may range from a nagging question about a health problem to an acute emergency like a heart attack or stroke. He or she comes into physical contact with a physician. The physician conducts an examination, asks questions about the problem, then (usually) takes some action to manage the uncertainty and charges a fee for the service.

For command of a vital knowledge base, American physicians have been able to charge several hundred billion dollars a year in what economists call "rent." As with most economically lucrative transactions, the doctor-patient relationship has been steeply asymmetrical relative to knowledge and, therefore, power.

By contrast, the resources on which consumers drew to frame their encounter with the physician were not terribly rich. What one could learn from one's family, friends, neighbors, schools, culture, and the popular press (for decades, *Reader's Digest* has been a widely read resource for consumer health information) essentially exhausted the available sources of medical knowledge. As late as

1998, women were more likely to get their medical information from media sources such as television, newspapers, and magazines than from physicians.[4]

THE TRADITIONAL CONSUMER EXPERIENCE OF HEALTHCARE

One does not have to search too long in one's recent memory of personal healthcare experiences to realize how cumbersome the health system is to use. Because it is difficult or impossible to reach most physicians by telephone or e-mail, most people must make an appointment to communicate with their physician. The gap between wanting medical knowledge and actually seeing the physician may range from days to weeks. For reasons explored in Chapter 4, this time lag could increase rather than diminish in the next decade as physicians of all specialties become increasingly scarce and difficult to see.

To see the physician, the consumer must take time off work, as physicians typically see patients during working hours. If the problem is with a child, the parent must take time off work and take the child out of school to meet the appointment. The time taken off work or out of school is a significant cost to the patient or family member, as well as to employers, that is not entered into account in the national health expenditures. If the physician practices in an urban or suburban setting, the consumer then may get stuck in traffic and may need to allow time for parking. Then they wait, often for minutes, but sometimes for hours, in the physician's office. Afterward, they get their eight minutes with the physician.

Depending in major part on the consumer's educational level, the actual question that brought him or her to the physician in the first place may or may not get asked; if asked, the answer may or may not be understood. In a 1997 *New York Times* consumer survey, 51 percent of women left the physician's office with unanswered questions. For women with less than a high school degree, fully 65 percent left the office with unanswered questions. Some 56 percent felt that physicians talked down to them some or most of the time.[5] The consumer will leave with a prescription or two, of which as many as 10 to 15 percent may never get filled, let alone used properly. In a couple of weeks, a bill arrives, which is frequently incorrect, requiring further interaction with the physician's office or the health plan.

THE IMPACT OF SYSTEMIC FAILURES ON PATIENTS AND FAMILIES

When complex medical problems arise, consumers and their families are all too often left to fend for themselves in a highly complex, poorly coordinated care framework. Shortly before he died of cancer, Avedis Donebedian, an eminent academic physician who pioneered the study of quality of healthcare, commented on his care experience at a large, distinguished academic health center:

> . . . there are areas where no one takes responsibility, where planning is weak, where I am left on my own. . . . the hospital floors are a disaster. I saw so many part-time nurses working variable hours. They come and go. Often, I couldn't tell whether I was dealing with a nurse, a technician, an attending physician or an attendant. I saw rampant discontinuity in nursing care. . . .

He went on to say, "The idea that patients should be involved in their care is not really practiced in a responsible way. Today people talk about patient autonomy, but it often gets translated into patient abandonment."[6]

In an impassioned critique of his wife's care at a world renowned East Coast teaching hospital, another expert on medical quality, Dr. Donald Berwick, compared the breakdown in teamwork (and the consequent shifting of the crushing responsibility for ensuring continuity of care to family members) to the Norman MacLean story, "Young Men and Fire."[7] MacLean chronicled the death of 13 smoke jumpers in the mountains in Montana during the 1949 fire season. According to MacLean, the young smoke jumpers died because they could not function as a team under the pressure of a sudden cataclysmic firestorm.

In Berwick's narrative, his wife, who suffered from a mysterious and potentially lethal spinal cord infection, was exposed to repeated mortal risk in the care process because crucial information on her health was not available to the clinical team taking care of her and because of continuous shifting of responsibility for making lifesaving care decisions. Berwick's repeated intervention was needed to provide the continuity and common sense the care system lacked,[8] despite the hospital's state-of-the-art, computerized electronic patient record system.

The not-surprising result of these problems is that consumer satisfaction with the health system experience is on a downward trend, as it is for notoriously customer-unfriendly sectors such as the airlines and insurance. The reality is that the logistics of medical care do not work for many American consumers, whether they simply need information about their health or require lifesaving care. The failure to manage the complexity of medicine and to care for people in a thoughtful and compassionate way has contributed to an emerging consumer revolt against medical institutions.

ORIGINS OF THE CONSUMER REVOLT AGAINST THE HEALTH SYSTEM

The consumer revolt against the present medical care system began during the late 1960s. The "shot heard round the world" in women's health was fired in 1970, when the Women's Health Book Collective of Boston published a "user's manual" for a woman's body entitled *Our Bodies, Ourselves.* Since its initial publication, it has been translated into 20 languages and has sold more than 4.5 million copies, making it by far the best-selling book ever published on health issues.

In strident and confident tones, *Our Bodies* urges women to take responsibility for their own health and to confront what was then (but is no longer) a largely male cadre of obstetricians/gynecologists and other physicians in determining how medical care is defined and delivered. This was at a time when only 7 percent of practicing obstetricians/gynecologists in the United States were women, according to the American Medical Association.[9]

This book helped embolden a generation of women to demand of their obstetricians/gynecologists options for childbirth and women's health concerns. It encouraged women to reject the surgical trappings of hospital-based childbirth in favor of a more natural approach. Many older, male obstetricians bridled at the large numbers of demanding "new women" who came to their appointment with typed lists of exactly how they wanted their care (and their babies!) to be delivered.

THE INTERNET: THE NEXT PHASE OF CONSUMERISM

A major engineering feat of the nineteenth century was to reverse the flow of the Chicago River and carry disease-producing human waste away from Chicago's lakefront. In a major feat of twentieth century engineering, the Internet reversed the centuries-old flow of health information. Thanks to the Internet, health information now flows "backward" from consumers to physicians. The Internet has enabled those people who are newly diagnosed with complex health problems to reach the scientific sources of information about their condition before their own time-famished physicians can (Figure 5.2).

Little did the visionary Department of Defense planners who conceived the Internet in the late 1960s understand that they were also creating a powerful weapon for women in their struggle with the

Figure 5.2: Knowledge Transmission in Medicine, Today

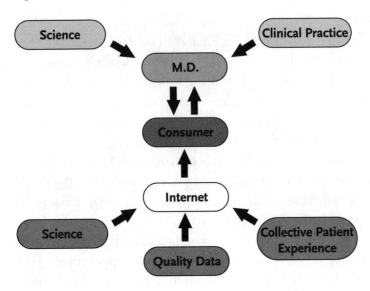

Source: Health Futures, Inc.

American health system. Indeed, few in Congress understood that by opening the Internet to public use in the Telecommunications Act of 1993, accessing health information would quickly become one of the most important uses of this powerful new tool.

Seeking health information is one of the most prevalent reasons why consumers log on to the Internet. On any given day, six million Americans can be found on the World Wide Web searching for health information. More Internet users have sought health information (62 percent) than have shopped online (61 percent), looked up stock quotes (42 percent), or checked sports scores (44 percent).[10] Furthermore, according to the Pew Trust, 47 percent of consumers who used the Internet reported that the information they found affected their decisions about the care they used.[11]

However, the Internet has done much more than democratize access to scientific knowledge. It is helping consumers select physicians based on feedback from their existing patients. Eventually, it will also help patients select hospital-based clinical programs and specialists based on their performance (morbidity and complication rates, infections, clinical volumes, years in practice, credentials, malpractice history, etc.). Most importantly, it helps give consumers and their families access to the collective wisdom and experience of others who are coping with and learning about a particular medical problem. As Howard Rheingold has written, the Internet enables "virtual communities" to convene around issues of common interest.[12] These communities represent loci of shared learning, as well as intellectual and emotional support, for those struggling with acute or chronic illness.

These community-creating effects extend well beyond the health system. A recent *New York Times* article documented that the Internet has contributed to a remarkable improvement in the recovery rate for missing children. The recovery rate has jumped from 62 percent in 1989 to 93 percent in 2002. The improvement is more astounding in those cases where the child is kidnapped by a non-family member. Before 1990, the recovery rate for these cases was around 35 percent; it increased to about 90 percent in 2002.[13]

The need to make sense of a life-changing event, like a cancer diagnosis, is the intangible element that keeps the consumer coming back to medical Internet. Some take the "Just the facts, Ma'am" approach and use the Internet to gather facts about their condition and what to do about it. Others are searching for referral information, answering questions such as, "Where is the best place for me to go to resolve my problem?" Yet others are searching for emotional support, whether as actual sufferers from the disease or as family members trying to help a stricken loved one. However consumers may use it, the advent of the Internet has shifted power in medicine from one-on-one relationships controlled by professionals to spontaneous, geographically dispersed networks that may include as many as 100,000 participants.

Several years ago, I had dinner with a Connecticut internist who recounted a "primal encounter" with this new healthcare consumer. Still shell-shocked from his interaction, this Yale-trained internist related that he had diagnosed a long-time patient with a dreadful rare, systemic, and fatal autoimmune disease that he had never encountered in his practice and had scheduled a treatment planning session with the now-terrified patient to begin addressing her problem.

The patient came to the meeting with a two-inch thick binder of articles she had downloaded via the Internet from national and international medical journals. The binder was tabbed for each organ system in the body affected by the disease. It also contained a basic science section on the potential genetic and molecular basis of the illness.

The patient placed the binder on the internist's desk and said, "Why don't we start here?" To extend the reversal of power, she added, "Did you know that one of your colleagues here in town has begun doing photodynamic therapy for my condition? Do you think I ought to see him?" As was most of the material in the binder, this was news to the physician, who took the encounter with wondering good nature.

When I related this story at one of my presentations, a physician posed the following rhetorical question about the exchange: "Why should I read it [the binder]? I'm only getting $30 for the visit and I just don't have time!" This response elicited gasps of disbelief from the nonphysicians in the audience. As I have subsequently learned, however, this response from physicians is not an unusual one.

The "why should I read it" response reflects at least two kernels of truth wrapped in a thick layer of barely examined and ugly emotions. True enough, many physicians do not feel they have enough time to do their jobs properly; and certainly, a lot of the material in the binder may not have been directly relevant to the treatment planning task at hand. It was, after all, assembled by a layperson without scientific training.

Remember, however, that the physician in Connecticut was dealing with a disease he had not treated before and thus needed to research the matter himself to participate meaningfully in the process. So what the patient did for the Connecticut physician was, in reality, helpful. In business, this process is called "outsourcing to the customer," which is what Federal Express did when it set up its web site to enable a customer to locate a package without going through its call center.

By taking the initiative, the *patient,* not the doctor, took charge of defining medical reality. In the Connecticut example, the physician did not explicitly delegate this task. Rather, the patient "volunteered," in a desperate effort to begin immediately the task of defining her own medical reality and options. The binder represented dozens of hours of tedious review of tens of thousands of page matches, reading, book marking, and downloading.

What the angry physician responder also missed was that, however well armed with information, the patient still engaged her physician and relied on his judgment. Physicians do not disappear from the equation. Rather, their dialog with a growing number of better-informed patients and family members will simply begin at a higher level of knowledge (or uncertainty) about the disease and its treatment options. The Internet is making the role of physician as teacher more explicit and eventually, as we will see in Chapter 8, more efficient.

The emotional subtext of the physician's anger is the feeling that their professional expertise is no longer respected. Whatever other pressures they may feel as members of one of the nation's most successful and prestigious professions, many physicians feel marginalized by many of the changes that took place in our healthcare system during the past 20 years.

The diminution of professional authority brought about by the Internet is not exclusive to medicine. Michael Lewis' recent book

Next explored the jarring invasion of professional space in law, investing and other disciplines by uncredentialed teenage Internet buffs. All knowledge-based professions face the same Internet-spawned leveling of knowledge gradients as medicine.[14]

ACCOMODATING DIFFERENT PERSPECTIVES

Consumers and patients differ in their needs, beliefs, and cultural values about their health. Accommodating these differences will be an important feature of tomorrow's health system. Many consumers will continue to want the old-style physician-patient relationship and do not wish to be bothered by the rigors of custom-fabricating their own knowledge base. Consumer research has found that some people will want to delegate as much responsibility as possible to their physicians (and perhaps then sue them if things do not work out as they wish). These patients, who rely solely on their physicians for health information, are described as "accepting." Approximately 8 percent of patients fall into this category.[15]

What patients and their families are really seeking, therefore, is not merely information, or even knowledge. They are really looking for *wisdom*—the thoughtful application of relevant medical knowledge to their unique situation. While Internet tools will certainly accelerate the flow of medical knowledge, converting that knowledge to wisdom will remain the physician's burden and responsibility.

Although their relationship sometimes contains adversarial elements, physicians and their patients/consumers share two common goals. First, they are united in seeking new knowledge. Both physicians and consumers are hungry for knowledge that will help lead to better care decisions. Second, and most important, they are both aligned in wanting to resolve the medical problem that brought them together. Finding the knowledge to do this represents the intersection of these goals.

CREATING A USER-FRIENDLY INFORMATION RESOURCE

The Internet is a popular knowledge resource, but it is also maddeningly difficult for many consumers to use. Moving from the present state of the medical Internet to a consumer-friendly knowledge resource is going to take a lot of work and will involve the efforts of practitioners and healthcare executives, as well as consumers. The following is a look at the current situation; later, we will take a look at the future.

Currently, the medical Internet is a bewildering mud slide of undifferentiated facts, opinions, pharmaceutical and health provider infomercials, personal web pages constructed by individual patients, bulletin boards and chat rooms hosted by volunteer physicians, scientific literature, press releases, and gossip. As of this writing, more than 20,000 health-related web sites could be found on the Internet,[16] and more than 12 million citations appear in the National Library of Medicine's MEDLINE service, available to consumers through its PubMed link.

A recent cursory effort to research lupus through the Yahoo! search engine yielded 848,000 page matches for a disease that affects only 500,000 Americans. In addition to all of these sources, I even found articles about wolves (the species is *Canus lupus*). Of course, if I had just been diagnosed with lupus, which is incurable, my motivation to wade through this information would have more than matched the logistical challenge.

The variable quality of medical information on the Internet is a widely acknowledged problem for anyone who uses it. One witty observer likened the current state of the medical Internet to a "virtual Haight/Ashbury." (For younger readers, the Haight/Ashbury was the district in San Francisco that spawned the hippie movement in the 1960s. Besides being a site of colorful street theater, it was also an open-air drug bazaar, where one could buy pills of dubious provenance from complete strangers and take one's chances.)

Indeed, consumer backlash against the Internet's mud slide of medical information could be detected as early as 2001. According to Harris Interactive, consumers are losing confidence in the Internet as a leverage point in their relationship to the medical care system (Figure 5.3). Despite the many millions invested in healthcare web sites, the medical Internet is daunting and difficult for many consumers to use.

A free market economist would point out that the highly variable quality of medical information on the Internet can be attributed to the fact that the information is supposed to be "free." A powerful social norm of the Internet is that intellectual property ought to be free and freely available to anyone who needs it. If it is true that "you get what you pay for," the fact that people have been unwilling to pay for medical information on the Internet has diminished the incentives to create accessible and reliable content and for people with proprietary knowledge to post it.

However, despite the logistical problems, when consumers confront a life-changing illness, the Internet is the principal destination postdiagnosis.[17] Logging on and commencing a search is an overt act of joining a community of inquiry and support for a specific problem. Clearly, consumers are going to need help, in addition to that of their physicians, in sorting through all of the potential knowledge domains about a given disease to find the "good stuff"—access to state-of-the-science knowledge and the treatment protocols that are testing that knowledge on the task of curing the disease.

CONSUMER POWER

During the 1980s and early 1990s, employers and the federal government experimented with delegating responsibility for managing healthcare to private health plans. Ambitious "health reform" proposals, such as those of the early Clinton administration, sought to shift responsibility for deciding what medical care was needed from doctors and patients to health plans. Buried in this idea was

Figure 5.3: Consumer Backlash

The Internet helped in:	1999 %	2001 %	Change %
Understanding of own health problems	73	55	−18
Managing personal health care overall	60	40	−20
Communications with doctor	51	31	−20
Compliance with treatments recommended by doctor	46	31	−15

Source: Harris Interactive. 2001. *Strategic Health Perspectives 2001.* Rochester, NY: Harris Interactive.

a strong element of medical paternalism—an assumption, which seems breathtakingly naive in retrospect, that ordinary citizens would permit their health needs to be defined for them by complete strangers with an economic interest in limiting their care.

The American public roundly rejected this idea. Acting through their elected representatives and the news media, consumers told the health system that *they* wanted to be the architects of their own care and definers of their own needs and not delegate that responsibility to hospital systems, health plans, employers, or the government. Indeed, the health plans that prospered during the 1990s were those, such as Blue Cross plans and preferred provider organizations (PPOs), that permitted consumers to continue relationships with hospitals and doctors they trusted and that had met their needs in the past.

If the first phase of the consumer movement in healthcare culminated in the rejection of external management of healthcare by health plans, the second phase will be the presentation of the bill. Health costs are presently exploding, and the cessation of supervision by health plans has contributed to that explosion.[18] Wide-open networks and unfettered access to services and technology, including new drugs, are expensive and have been a major factor in the present acceleration of health costs after nearly a decade of relative calm.

Consumer choice as an organizing principal in healthcare will prove very expensive, as the new cost-management technologies giving consumers the choice they have demanded while holding hospitals, doctors, pharmaceutical companies, and others accountable for efficient use of money have yet to be accepted.

THE CONSUMER INFORMATION MODEL OF THE FUTURE

What consumers need is help organizing medical knowledge relative to their health and the relevant care options. The "heavy lifting" in this process will be done by the intelligent clinical software discussed in Chapter 2 that hospitals and physicians will use to manage their clinical encounters with patients (Figure 5.4). Rather than physicians and hospitals hoarding the decision-support capabilities in their clinical software, consumers will demand and gain access to the same rules engines and documentation their caregivers use. Those who design this software must accommodate the reality that consumers will need access to this crucial knowledge and that it will inevitably be used as a teaching tool by physicians and other caregivers.

In addition, automated search engines, called "intelligent agents," will assist physicians and consumers in winnowing the vast amount of potential information into the subset of relevant information that informs specific decisions for particular patients. These engines will become far more efficient as the computer mark-up language XML spreads in medicine.

Furthermore, established medical institutions—medical schools such as Harvard and Johns Hopkins, multispecialty clinics such as the Mayo Clinic, national medical entities such as the American Medical Association, and specialty clinical societies like the American College of Cardiology—will compete to function as "trusted sources" of medical knowledge. These institutions will rely on the wisdom and judgment of their physicians to identify the subset of

Figure 5.4: Knowledge Transmission in Medicine, Twenty-first Century

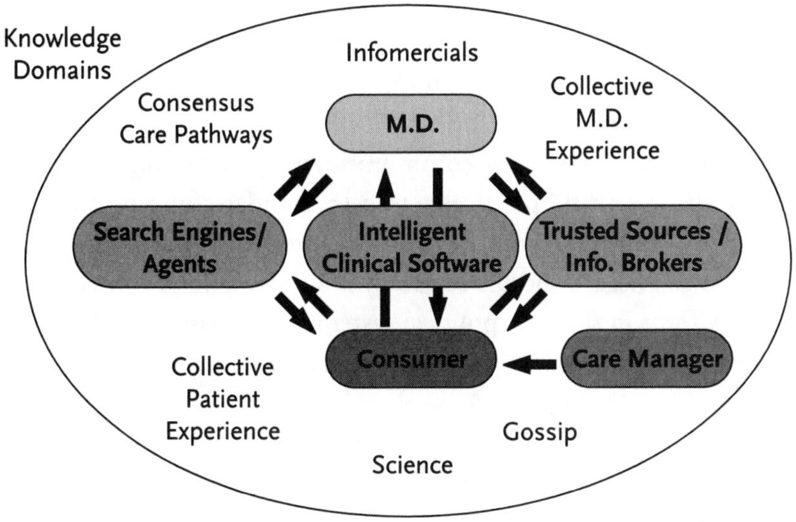

Source: Health Futures, Inc.

information about specific diseases that patients should know and trust. The Mayo Clinic began working toward providing accessible consumer health information in the early 1990s with its pioneering (and outstanding) CD-ROM and was an early and formidable Internet presence with its Oasis web site.

Both automated and person-assisted searches will help consumers narrow the uncertainty associated with present medical Internet use and appreciably cut the time and cost of acquiring information. Although present search tools such as Google are free to the user and subsist largely on advertising revenues and marketing tie-ins, the next generation of search tools will operate on a subscription basis, as the most successful consumer web sites such as ConsumerReports.com do today.

The Internet will also enable virtual communities focused on specific diseases to function as full-fledged social institutions, with communications, advocacy, and logistical assistance for consumers and their families. Communities of disease sufferers, comprising patients and their families, providers, health insurers, and vendors of various kinds, will use web-based software to raise funds for purchasing medical consultation on their own or evaluate referrals to hospitals or specialists with unique capabilities for treating the disease of interest.

Virtual disease-specific communities will also be able to use web tools for organizing political action to mandate funding coverage of their conditions by federal and employer-based health insurance programs. Disease-specific advocacy is already a major, and controversial, force in the U.S. political system, as successes in publicizing breast cancer and AIDS research agendas have demonstrated.

CONTINUOUS ACCESS TO KNOWLEDGE: E-HEALTH'S PROMISE TO CONSUMERS

The question begged by all the progress in IT for consumers is, why can't IT shorten and sharpen the search for medical knowledge and strengthen the doctor-patient relationship at the same time? It can, and it will. Broadband connectivity, intelligent clinical software, and Internet search utilities can help alleviate what Don Berwick has called "the tyranny of the visit" and herald a new, "always on" relationship between physicians and those they care for.

Information technology will not only enable physicians and patients to be connected and to communicate asynchronously 24 hours a day, but it will also permit clinical information to be gathered and evaluated from the consumer's study, as in the David Sandy example at the beginning of this book, and the physician's home. Any two points that can be connected (by wire, fiber, or wireless connection) can serve as surrogates for the physician's exam room or even the hospital room.

Physicians can forward articles, illustrations, and other information to patients before and after physical meetings, instead of receiving binders of photocopied articles from patients at the time of the visit.[19] Information can flow both ways continuously.

Intelligent clinical software can help physicians stratify those they take care of into risk groups and launch outbound calls to find out how their patients are, whether they are taking their medication, and whether the medication is having the desired effect (or undesired adverse effects). Often, the people who present the real problem are those not in contact with the physician but who need to be. Information technology can enable physicians to be in continuous contact with their entire practice panels, not merely those who identify themselves as "sick" at a given moment.

Instead of being constrained to visit the physician or be admitted to an institution, consumers can subscribe to a physician's services, just as they subscribe to broadband or cable. Instead of using doctors' office staffs and nurses to joust continuously with health plans over payment and pharmacy benefits management companies over prescription renewals, physicians' office staff will help "program" the physician's information channel, monitor and evaluate the flow of patient communications, grade them for urgency, and schedule needed visits or treatments, or intervene on the physician's behalf to answer questions or resolve problems.

Face-to-face or voice-to-voice communication is essential in some situations, like documenting initial history, performing physicals, or making diagnoses, but these encounters can be strengthened by prior electronic interchanges. The personal touch in medicine will never disappear, but eliminating the unnecessary or poorly prepared contacts will create more time to lengthen and deepen the face-to-face part of medicine, as well as save patients and family members wasted time.

Those who pay for care must be willing to sponsor such relationships. Physicians have legitimate concerns about not being compensated for electronic contact with patients. Although some health plans are experimenting with "fee for e-health" consultation payment structures, a more reliable and cost-effective method of paying for these services will be as part of a global fee or subscription. As asserted later, the health plan's role should be to sponsor relationships between physicians and consumers, not to intervene and structure them.

CONCLUSION

As access to knowledge about health becomes more democratized and widespread, power will continue shifting to consumers in the American health system. This shift is as powerful and irresistible as an earthquake. Not all parts of the health system will be able to cope with this tectonic shift, and some pieces of the old knowledge franchise will crumble. As we will see later, empowering consumers and making it easier to use the health system is the most important way hospitals, doctors, and health plans can use this powerful new toolbox of Internet applications.

NOTES

1. National Center for Health Statistics. 2001. "Utilization of Ambulatory Medical Care by Women: United States, 1997–98." Series Report 13, No. 149.

2. Boston Women's Health Book Collective. 1998. *Our Bodies, Ourselves.* New York: Simon and Schuster.

3. Weber, D. O. 1999. "Men's Health: The Last Great Frontier." *Healthcare Strategist* 3 (10): 1–8.

4. Elder, J. 1997. "Poll Finds Women are the Health-Savvier Sex, and the Warier." *New York Times*, June 22.

5. Ibid.

6. Donebedian, A. 2001. "A Founder of Quality Assessment Encounters a Troubled System Firsthand. Interview by Fitzhugh Mullan." *Health Affairs* 20 (1): 137–41.

7. MacLean, N. 1992. *Young Men and Fire.* Chicago: University of Chicago Press.

8. Berwick, D. 1999. "Escape Fire." Plenary Address to the 7th Annual Forum on Quality Improvement in Healthcare.

9. Pasko, T., B. Seidman, and S. Birkhead. 1982. *Physician Characteristics and Distribution in the US*. Chicago: AMA Press.

10. Pew Internet & American Life Project Tracking surveys. March 2000–present "Internet Activities." [Online information; retrieved 12/09/02.] http://www .pewinternet.org/reports/chart.asp?img=Interne7.htm.

11. Fox, S., and L. Rainie. 2000. "The Online Healthcare Revolution: How the Web is Helping Americans Take Better Care of Themselves." Washington, DC: Pew Trust Internet American Life Project.

12. Rheingold, H. 1993. *The Virtual Community: Homesteading on the Electronic Frontier*. Cambridge, MA: MIT Press.

13. Lee, J. 8. 2002. "Lost to Found, With Technology's Help." *New York Times*, April 25.

14. Lewis, M. 2001. *Next: The Future Just Happened*. New York: Norton.

15. Taylor, H., and R. Leitman. 2001. "The Increasing Impact of eHealth on Consumer Behavior." *Harris Interactive* 1 (21): 1–9.

16. Health and Pharma Insight Newsletter. 2002. "Ask the Expert." Manhattan Research, LLC. [Online information; retrieved 12/17/02.] http://www .manhattanresearch.com/newsletter1202.htm.

17. Ibid. Fox, S., and L. Rainie.

18. Center for Studying Health System Change. "Community Tracking Study: Physician Survey." [Online information; retrieved 12/30/02.] http://www.hschange .com/index.cgi?data=04.

19. T. Ferguson. 2002. "e-Patients, Online Health, and the Search for Sustainable Healthcare: A Guide for Grantmakers." Working Paper. Princeton, NJ: The Robert Wood Johnson Foundation.

CHAPTER 6

Health Plans

As THIS BOOK was being written, no segment of American healthcare is under greater stress than its private health insurance system. A decade ago, the promise of managed care seemed bright enough for the Clinton administration to bet most of its political capital on using managed care as a cornerstone of health reform. Managed care advocates not only believed that their plans could arrest wildly escalating health costs, but also assumed that they could redress income inequities in the healthcare professions, reduce excess capacity in the hospital system, and actually improve people's health.

However, by the end of the decade, managed health plans dwelt in the societal doghouse, along with the tobacco and oil companies, due not only in part to unrealistic expectations but also to poor execution, arrogance, dreadful customer service, and a relentlessly hostile press.[1] Health plans found few defenders in the court of public opinion or the political system, despite high rates of satisfaction of their members, extraordinarily skilled political advocates in Washington, and nearly a decade of relief from rising health costs.[2]

The financial recovery of health plans from the catastrophic operating losses they experienced during the late 1990s makes it possible to address the larger issue of repositioning health insurance as a business, as well as renovating its public image. Leveraging innovation in information technology, particularly Internet connectivity, holds the key to the revival of these firms. Major health insurance functions—network development and management, enrollment and eligibility verification, medical claims submission and payment, and medical management—become not only more transparent and affordable but more politically acceptable through use of Internet applications.

Information technology is likely to make a more visible difference in health insurance than any other area of healthcare through about 2010. Digitizing core health insurance functions could not only lower the amount of the health insurance premium devoted to overhead, but also markedly improve customer service, a major weakness of many health plans. Whether the plans can accomplish this conversion and embrace the new business model remains to be seen, but this chapter discusses promising innovations to assist that conversion.

COPING WITH GROWTH BADLY

The number of enrollees in managed care plans almost quadrupled during the 1990s, and many health plans were completely overwhelmed by enrollment growth. The computer systems of these plans were, in many cases, completely incapable of "scaling up" to manage the tens of millions of new managed care subscribers.

As a result, many plans' information systems broke down, resulting in lengthy delays in paying providers, long waits for customer service on claims, and tangle-footed bureaucratic interference in the medical care process. The cause of the systems failures in health plans was fairly obvious: a depressing fraction of payment transactions were (and still are) driven by manual paper processing and telephone interactions. A single health plan, Humana, receives some

20 million telephone calls annually from its members, each of which costs $3 to answer.[3]

The sheer volume and complexity of transactions in the American health financing system boggles the mind. The vast majority of healthcare is paid for test by test, visit by visit, hospital stay by hospital stay. The result in 2000 was 5.1 billion actual claims for payment, and tens of billions of other interactions (referral authorizations, eligibility verifications, etc.) between providers and health insurers processed *manually* by an army of clerks.[4] According to Faulkner and Gray, only 18 percent of all HMO claims and 45 percent of all commercial health insurance claims were even submitted electronically in 1999.[5] The vast majority of these claims must be processed manually because they are incomplete or have inconsistent data.[6]

The inability of health plans to harness IT effectively has been a critical strategic weakness of these companies. For example, the failure of its information systems to cope with rapid enrollment growth played a crucial role in the near-collapse of Oxford Health Plan in 1998 and of the Harvard Pilgrim Health Plan in 1999. Despite the obvious incentives to upgrade their information systems, investment by managed care firms lags far behind other information-intensive sectors of the economy.

According to Gartner, health insurers spent only 3.4 percent of their gross revenues in 1999 on IT, compared with 4.1 percent for telecommunications firms and 6.1 percent for financial services. (Hospitals have historically spent even less, about 2.5 percent.[7])

Moreover, when health plans get into financial trouble, innovative IT strategies are often sacrificed to the budget cutter's sharp knife. When Foundation Health Plan's operating profit disappeared during 1998, one of the first casualties was its promising Fourth Generation Medical Management System, which combined innovative call-center operations with physician connectivity through personal digital assistants and other portable computing devices.

CREATING EFFICIENT HEALTH PLANS

E-commerce

In other sectors of the economy, the movement to e-commerce has had a common set of effects: marked reductions in transaction costs, increased speed of both transactions and the flow of cash related to them, increased transparency of the value chain and the customer service process, and vanishing margins of traditional intermediaries such as dealers, brokers, and wholesalers. [8]

If these effects manifest themselves in health insurance, 70 to 90 percent unit-cost reductions are expected by digitizing these functions and performing them through network computing: claims processing, subscriber enrollment and verification (e.g., "Are you covered?"), medical management (e.g., "Is the medical care appropriate and covered?"), network management (e.g., managing all the contracts with hospitals and doctors), and an array of related administrative functions (collecting insurance premiums from employers, regulatory compliance, etc.).

The expenses associated with these activities claim anywhere from 10 to 20 percent of the health insurance premium, and are deducted from the health insurer's cash flow before physicians or hospitals receive a dime of payment for their services. The management consulting firm Booz-Allen and Hamilton has estimated the distribution, consultation, and administrative expenses of private health insurance in the United States in 1999 at $18 billion per year: $5 billion for sales and marketing costs (principally commissions to insurance brokers), $3 billion to benefits consultants who manage health insurance contracting for employers, and $10 billion for health plan administrative overhead. [9]

INTERNET RELIEF FROM THE PAPER AVALANCHE

Liberating employers, health plans, and consumers from the blizzard of paperwork surrounding healthcare is the most compelling and most immediate opportunity offered by the Internet. A study by Ernst & Young (now Cap Gemini Ernst & Young) estimated that health insurers could reduce their overhead expenses by $3.6 billion, or more than one-third, by incorporating e-commerce solutions.[10] These cost reductions could greatly improve the business operations of health plans, as well as their profitability. More important, however, digitizing their operations could markedly improve customer service and thus improve the firms' public image.

Processing medical claims electronically predates the Internet by more than 20 years. A surprisingly large percentage of health claims already flow to health insurers through electronic conduits. In 2000, of the 5.1 billion medical claims processed by public and private health insurers in the United States, 67 percent were transmitted electronically, primarily through computer tapes and high-bandwidth dedicated telephone lines like T1 lines.[11]

More than 86 percent of all hospital claims and 89 percent of all pharmacy claims were transmitted electronically in 2000. Unfortunately, tape submission, the dominant mode of transmittal, is not interactive and frequently results in a lengthy paper exchange to correct errors and omissions as well as delays in payment. The cost of adjudicating a "dirty" health insurance claim increases from less than a dollar for a "clean claim" to as much as $50 per claim.

Far greater savings are likely to be achieved by moving the billions of other healthcare transactions that do not directly involve medical payment to interactive broadband and markedly improving the quality and accuracy of the claims themselves.[12] The nonclaims transactions, which number in the tens of billions annually, include verifying eligibility, determining if a specific health service is covered, and authorizing referrals or hospitalizations.

What the Internet adds to electronic commerce in healthcare is an open, public infrastructure that enables health plans to connect to physicians and consumers who cannot afford a T1 line. It is not the state of Internet technology that is preventing physicians' offices or consumers in their homes from tracking the status of a medical claim. It is the state of the health plan's software and the lack of standardization of information requests by payers that holds the industry back, as well as the failure of physicians to automate their billing and clinical information functions, as discussed in Chapter 5.

Affordable connectivity is available for health plans to connect to consumers and physicians through the Internet. Health insurers are working overtime to reprogram their information systems to make this connectivity possible. Doing this will relieve their overburdened call centers of huge volumes of unnecessary telephone calls and enable customers to answer many questions about their coverage or payment for care themselves.

As mentioned earlier, physicians' accounts receivable and clerical costs could be markedly reduced if their claims could be filed, evaluated, and paid electronically, with the patient's portion of the cost charged to his or her credit card. The technology to make the medical payment transaction as simple as the credit card transaction to purchase a shirt is already available. Reprogramming health plans' information systems to accept electronic inquiries and teaching consumers and physician office staffs to use the tools is the big barrier, along with the aforementioned lack of consistency in data needs by the payers.

HIPAA'S IMPACT

The federal government actually helped the cause for simpler transactions when Congress passed the Health Insurance Portability and Accountability Act of 1996 (HIPAA). The principal purpose of this law was to make it easier for employees to retain insurance coverage when they changed employment, as well as to protect the confidentiality and security of electronic transmission of personal medical information.

A much overlooked feature of this legislation, however, was that it requires health insurers to use a common clinical coding scheme and common formats for electronic medical claims and other medical transactions. The Administrative Simplification provisions of

HIPAA have catalyzed what will eventually amount to tens of billions of dollars in IT upgrades by health insurers, hospitals, and others to reprogram their computer systems to use these common formats.

These mandated expenditures were not welcome news for the managers of health plans, because HIPAA arrived as their cash flow departed. Notably, the HIPAA mandates coincided with a virtual freeze in federal Medicare payments to hospitals and health insurers. HIPAA was a classic example of an "unfunded mandate"—a government action that increases costs without commensurate funds to pay them. (Indeed, pressures from the health insurance industry, notably Blue Cross plans, led Congress to enact a one-year delay in implementing these provisions late in their 2001 session.)

The federal government can legitimately be criticized for not appropriating funds to help physicians, hospitals, and health plans make these needed systems changes mandated by HIPAA. By not allocating funds, the government has increased health costs for everyone, not just for government-funded patients. Having said this, however, the likelihood is that the systems conversions HIPAA requires will save billions of dollars in operating costs for health plans and providers by accelerating the movement to paperless payment. [13]

However much they might complain about the government telling them how to run their businesses, health plans would probably never have agreed to common formats for electronic claims filing on their own, because historically each has used its own formats and had little incentive to cooperate with competitors in reducing hospital and doctor overhead. Also, given the large capital expenditures involved, health plans would have delayed making these investments absent the federal mandate.

GETTING MANAGED CARE OUT OF THE EXAM ROOM

Medical management is the part of managed care that enraged consumers and physicians the most. Most consumers did not like the idea of a third party, stranger both to them and their physician, deciding what they needed. But this is precisely what employers hired health plans to do: eliminate care that enriched hospitals or doctors but was not actually needed by patients.

The health plan's medical director, aided by external consultants, traditionally made medical coverage decisions. These recommendations were usually based on the available scientific evidence of clinical effectiveness and the cost/benefit relationship for the plan and subscribers. Until relatively recently, these criteria were enforced by, literally, case-by-case authorization of nurses sitting in cubicles in Tucson or Omaha reading off computer screens.

This intrusive method of cost control, called prior authorization, was costly both for health plans and for health providers. It was also a tremendous political liability. Because it reduced physician and hospital incomes, it is not surprising that providers would mobilize to try and outlaw the practice.

Before they could do so, however, health insurers themselves began studying how much they saved by prior authorization and what it cost them. In 1999, one of the nation's largest health plans, United HealthGroup, abandoned case-by-case prior authorization for all but a handful of extremely costly services because it discovered that this practice was actually costing them more to do it than it saved.

This decision garnered tremendous positive publicity for United and for health plans generally, because it eliminated a major irritant in the relationship with both doctors and consumers. Many other health insurers have followed suit.[14] To make this transition possible, United and other health plans invested billions of dollars in automating claims processing and using expert systems to identify patterns of health services that strongly suggested fraud or economic abuse of patients.

The Internet will streamline and make much more transparent this key part of health plan operations—its supervision over medical care itself. As it migrates onto the Internet, medical management (that is, determining if the care a physician proposes is covered and appropriate) will become essentially invisible and instantaneous, embedded directly in electronic claims management.

Medical management will thus become an "exception review" process, as the flow of claims will be automatically monitored to identify physician or hospital practices that are inappropriate. Only a small number of very expensive procedures or services will require prior review by the health plan.

DEFINING THE HEALTH PLAN'S CUSTOMER

More fundamentally, however, health plans have begun to reexamine who their real customers are. The fundamental message of the managed care backlash to the health plans is that consumers and physicians would not tolerate the continued intrusion of a financially motivated third party in their relationship.

The fact that health plans worked for employers made it impossible to answer succinctly the question, who is the health plan's customer? Under "total replacement" coverage, the reality was that the consumer was often not a customer of the health plan at all, but rather its prisoner. Prisoners were referred to in actuarial jargon as "lives" and measured by the thousands.

The inability to answer clearly the question of who is the customer is often fatal to businesses. Technologies that people believe are being used by corporate enterprises to further their own economic interests almost inevitably become targets of political reaction. The reaction of consumers against genetically modified foods, which benefited farmers and agribusiness conglomerates, but not obviously the consumer herself, is a classic example.

Consumers as Sheep?

The problem of defining the consumer's role also afflicted the health policy proposals on which the Clinton administration gambled its presidency. An influential health policy group called the Jackson Hole Group, founded by Dr. Paul Ellwood (and which met in Dr. Ellwood's Jackson Hole, Wyoming, condominium), promoted managed care–based reform. The "hole" in the Jackson Hole Group's so-called "Consumer Choice Health Plan" was the role of the consumer. Most of the tinkering with tax policy and insurance regulation in the Jackson Hole proposals was aimed at compelling consumers to shop for health coverage with their grocery money. Consumers who wished more lavish coverage than a basic, standard benefit package would have been required to use their own money.

Once the consumer selected a health plan, however, his or her work was done. After selecting the health plan, according to the Jackson Hole proposal, consumers became little lambs, to be shepherded through the complexities of healthcare by "their" managed care plan. It was up to the managed care plan selected "voluntarily" by the consumer to decide what healthcare was appropriate and who should provide it, and we would all just say "baaaaaah" and go along.

Hindsight is always 20/20, but it seems breathtakingly naive in retrospect that health policymakers could assume that consumers (read "baby boom women in charge of their family's health") would surrender to shadowy medical directorates with a financial agenda the final say in decisions about what care they or their families needed, let alone who should provide it.

Under their version of managed care, Jackson Hole policy advocates assumed that medical decisions would ultimately be made by local physician groups themselves, not medical bureaucrats in some glass-fronted corporate office tower in Connecticut. The Jackson Holers did not foresee that the vast majority of growth in managed care would be gained through very broad networks where the health plans retained the ultimate decision-making authority about medical necessity for themselves, and continued paying doctors on a (discounted) fee basis.

As a result, many consumers got the worst of both worlds: no choice of health plan and corporate medicine managed (centrally and badly) by health plans overwhelmed by rapid enrollment growth. Deprived of a voice in selecting their health plan by total replacement coverage, consumers roared in the press and the political arena and helped catalyze a flood of state and federal consumer protection legislation.

DELIVERING VALUE FOR CONSUMERS

For reasons that will be explored more fully below, the employer's role in health benefits may diminish in future years. As it does, it will become clear that the real customer of the health plan is, and always was, the family, and its designated representative, the "woman in charge of her family's health." Creating and delivering measurable value for families is the only obvious way out of the health insurance industry's present political and economic problems. The emerging vision of "consumer-centric" health insurance is powered by IT.

Information technology, particularly Internet technology, can provide health plans multiple opportunities to create value for their real customers. These opportunities include the following:

- Helping consumers minimize the risk of poor-quality care
- Delivering disease-management content to high-risk patients
- Promoting informed choice through medical decision support software
- Offering consumers "do it yourself" network-development tools
- Creating customer service portals accessible through the web

Helping Consumers Minimize Risk

Most consumers are unaware that they may have as much as a fivefold variation in their risk of dying after a surgical procedure, depending on which surgical team or hospital they use or which community they get care in.[15] Indeed, this may be information that people do not *want* to know. Consumers naively assume that their physicians will refer them to the safest specialist or hospital. They do not realize that physicians tend to refer to their local colleagues and are pressured to admit patients to their local hospital, whether it is the safest place for care or not.

Hospitals have been profoundly uncomfortable with publicizing their own clinical track records, although in December 2002, a coalition of hospital groups committed to a common reporting format for clinical quality.[16] Because of the superheated litigation climate, hospitals and physicians have had a powerful incentive not to report their error rates. To avoid lawsuits, in fact, providers have a powerful incentive to cover up their mistakes, not to collaborate in reducing them. (For a superb history of why "quality" has not been a central issue in healthcare, read Michael Millenson's *Demanding Medical Excellence.*[17])

Health plans, however, have a powerful incentive to help their customers make better choices: medical errors are expensive, and health plans (as well as Medicare and Medicaid) pay the bill for them. Hospital-borne infections, readmissions after a procedure, anesthesia accidents, and medication errors all result in extra medical cost and suffering for patients.

Because consumers have reacted negatively to being told which doctors or hospitals to use, health plans have devised an alternate way of influencing consumer behavior: by creating quality "maps" of the health system. They publish hospital surgical mortality rates, infection rates, adverse drug reaction incidence, and consumer-satisfaction information on their web sites and encourage consumers to consult the sites before making a decision about where to receive care. Consumers who factor this information into their decisions will voluntarily select less risky programs. In doing so, they will not only save themselves from potential harm, but also save the health plan money in reduced health costs. By becoming advocates for consumer safety, health plans can assist their subscribers in making better decisions that affect their own health.

If the consumer's choice of safer programs saves the health plan money, it follows that reducing the amount of the patient's cost sharing if he or she selects the safest programs would be an effective way for health plans to focus consumer attention on the consequences of their decisions. Sharing the savings with consumers while preserving their freedom to choose where they go makes good economic sense.

Health plans can secure quality information by mining mortality and complication rate information from their trail of medical claims. It may be difficult to organize that information in a way that is statistically valid, but it is worth the effort. Sharing quality information across health plans would lead to better and more reliable estimates of actual quality. Pooling private insurance quality information with that of the federal agency that runs the Medicare program, the Centers for Medicare & Medicaid Services (CMS, the agency formerly known as the Health Care Financing Administration, or HCFA), would yield an even more formidable database (though one whose interpretation would be subject to violent objections by those organizations that do not fare well in the rankings or that have concerns about the methodology).

Employers are moving more aggressively along the quality front. Through an industry consortium called the Leapfrog Group, employers are encouraging their employees to consult the Leapfrog web site to identify local hospitals that meet quality standards. These standards include, tellingly, whether the hospital has computerized physician order entry, as well as more conventional standards related to the quality of staffing of intensive care units and service volumes, which correlate with better results (e.g., minimum number of open heart procedures per year).

Initially, Leapfrog is not going to abridge their employees' freedom of choice. They are not going to exclude from payment hospitals that do not meet these criteria from their health coverage. Rather, they will rely on voluntary decisions by consumers based on Leapfrog's comparative information. If hospital industry resistance thwarts voluntary measures, Leapfrog retains the option of excluding nonperforming hospitals from their panels or applying higher copayments to use their services.

Information technology—specifically expert systems in health plans and the federal government and Internet connectivity—is making it possible to systematize this process and make the results available to anyone who seeks them. Medical error variation is precisely the type of information consumers are seeking on the Internet.

Delivering Disease-management Content to High-risk Patients

Chronic disease is America's principal disease burden. Consumers who visit Internet health web sites are doing so in most cases for disease-specific information to help them cope with and manage the impact of these diseases on their lives.

Most chronic diseases are, by definition, incurable. Managing them to minimize their impact on the lives and livelihoods of their victims requires interaction between the sufferer and the health system. Each side of the physician-consumer relationship has a contribution to make to control the impact of the disease. The two principal costs in this process are the visit (to a physician's office, clinic, or emergency room) and the prescription. Both medical expenses are, to an impressive extent, controllable and at least partially avoidable. The consumer's own behavior is a major determinant of how avoidable medical expenses are.

Disease management evolved as a way to help physicians get their patients to do the things they needed to do to control their own disease risk. In the case of insulin-dependent diabetes, these actions are complex and involve monitoring blood sugar levels, precisely medicating themselves at the right time, managing their own diet and weight, and a host of smaller factors. If one lived with a physician, presumably one could be checked on these things continuously. However, because most diabetics do not live with physicians, continuous monitoring is awkward.

Short of periodic telephone contact (which is inexpensive), disease management either required nurses to visit the patient in the home and record health indicators (which is expensive) or else required the patient to visit a clinic and be evaluated (which is both time consuming and expensive). In IT jargon, the "user interface" for disease management was neither user friendly nor efficient.

With the advent of the Internet and affordable connectivity, disease management suddenly became far more efficient and easier to use. No one has a more powerful vested interest in making it work than health plans (and Medicare). What the Internet enables health plans to do is to connect 24/7 through a web site with their "frequent fliers"—chronically ill patients who are attempting to manage their diseases. Having connected to those patients, health plans can offer them interactive disease management software that enables patients to enter relevant clinical information, symptoms, and related items in a structured way and receive advice from the software, or from humans monitoring the software, about what to do next.

Evidence is emerging that patients love these interactions because they are convenient and responsive. In addition, there is compelling early evidence that the savings in reduced health costs (avoided visits to emergency rooms or hospitalizations) are substantial enough to justify giving computers to chronically ill people who do not have them and teaching them how to use them.[18]

Internet connectivity is not the only way in which health plans can connect to their chronically ill patients. Sophisticated voice-response technology, such as Eliza, mentioned earlier, can initiate outbound calls to check on patients' health status, confirm prescription drug use, check on renewals, and search for problems.

Promoting Informed Choice

If there was a core message in the managed care backlash, it was that consumers want to be the architects of their own care. Helping consumers make better, more informed choices is one way health plans can help create value for them.

A number of years ago, Dr. John Wennberg and his colleagues at Dartmouth College developed a medical decision support tool called Informed Choice for consumers newly diagnosed with a threatening medical condition for which multiple treatment options are available. Originally developed in an interactive, but logistically challenging, laser disc format (it is now in a web format and is markedly improved), Informed Choice guides a consumer and his or her physician through a sequence of questions that helps consumers identify their objectives in managing the disease.

Consumers are asked, for example, how sensitive they are to pain from a medical procedure, how much cost matters to them, and what degree of sacrifice in the quality of life they are willing to tolerate. The answers to these questions are factored into choosing what method of resolving the medical problem best fits the patient's needs.

Health plans should be interested in the Wennberg process and similar decision-support tools for two reasons. First, consumers who went through the Informed Choice process had significantly higher compliance rates for whatever treatment option they chose and were much more satisfied with the care they subsequently received. This should not surprise anyone; they participated actively in matching the chosen method of treatment to their own needs and thus "owned" the resulting choice.[19] Second, consumers who went through the process chose invasive forms of treatment like surgery much less often, significantly reducing the costs they incurred.

Offering Consumers Do-it-yourself Network Development Tools

For decades, health plans saw themselves as "aggregators" of care—bundling hospitals and doctors together into a single "transaction" for employers. For some consumers, the convenience outweighed the loss of choice involved. For many others, the interference with established relationships with hospitals and doctors represented an intolerable intrusion by the health plan into their lives. The Internet has given employers and health plans a powerful tool that enables the "mass customization" of networks to accommodate consumers' existing relationships with doctors and hospitals.

Indeed, some employers are going further by simply outsourcing choice of health plans and providers through what is called "defined contribution" health benefits. This approach is modeled on the 401(k) pension benefit, in which the employer funds the benefit, but the employee manages it, selecting the mutual fund or investments that best meet their financial objectives and needs. Under a defined-contribution health benefit, employers fund the benefit, but employees target it.

Using a personal web page, employers can give their employees a vehicle for placing themselves in a health plan, or, using a somewhat more radical approach, employees can select their own provider network (primary care physician, specialists, hospitals, pharmacies, etc.) and use an eBay-type auction site to negotiate payment rates with them.

A recently launched Internet health enterprise, Vivius, is helping employers and health plans bring this capability to employees. Working with health plans, Vivius provides employees a personal web page that enables them to select their own physicians based on their stated rates. There are no medical claims in Vivius' model. Rather, providers set their own per capita payment rate for individual consumer (that is, a monthly rate per consumer). This rate is adjusted automatically by Vivius software to reflect the age and sex of the patient.

After selecting the doctors and hospitals they wish to work with, Vivius adds the total cost of contracting with these physicians and compares it to the amount that the employer has contributed. The consumer then pays the difference on a credit card. The total amount the consumer pays in a year is capped, and a wrap-around indemnity insurance product, protecting the consumer from catastrophic medical expenses, funds costs above the cap. There are a number of companies in this "virtual" health plan market, with variations on this model, including Definity, Luminos, and Health-Market.[20]

Creating Consumer Service Portals

When health plans succeed in digitizing their core administrative operations, taking the next step—extending self-service capabilities to consumers through a web site—is relatively simple. If the claims trail becomes digital, it is possible for consumers to type in a security code and password and track the status of their medical claims. This is essentially the same process that Federal Express uses to enable consumers to track packages on the FedEx web site.

Consumers' personal health benefits web pages can be customized to help them select their own unique coverage and enable consumers to find out quickly if a service is covered and how much their share of the cost will be. It can also enable consumers to read the criteria the managed care plan used to decide if a service is covered and the process by which the plan arrived at its policy. Finally, the personal web site can be customized to deliver health information on issues particularly relevant to the consumer.

A common denominator of all of these consumer service opportunities for health plans is that, to some degree, they all involve "outsourcing" to the customer various functions formerly performed by the plan. The list of benefits from this practice is not insignificant: reducing medical risk; more efficiently fighting chronic disease; making better decisions about what care is needed; choosing doctors, hospitals, or benefit designs that meet the consumer's specific needs; absorbing some of the health plan's insurance risk (through defined-contribution care); and interacting with the health plan's administrative systems.

Consumers have demanded greater influence over these decisions. It is a powerful message that health plans are responding to by leveraging IT to enable consumers to do these things themselves.

DEFINED-CONTRIBUTION HEALTHCARE—
THE NEW, NEW THING?

Defined-contribution health coverage seems to make a lot of sense. Under a defined-contribution model, the employer no longer provides a health benefit, but merely provides employees a fixed amount of money to purchase health coverage. The employee-benefits precedent was set by 401(k) plans, which employers fund but employees manage.

Defined-contribution healthcare would certainly reinforce a powerful trend toward more consumer influence over healthcare. It *might* exert a braking influence on health cost growth. Removing the employer from the health plan selection decision also would help to clarify, once and for all, that the real customer of the health plan is the subscriber or family.

How practical is it to believe that it will replace conventional defined-benefit health insurance? Realistically, there are numerous practical barriers to its emergence as an alternative to traditional health insurance. These include employer and labor union resistance to abandoning defined-benefit coverage, affordability and cost discipline, risk selection, and provider resistance to assuming economic risk. It is also reasonable to assume that consumers will not voluntarily take on additional health cost exposure if they can avoid it.

In my view, premature obituaries have been written for the defined-benefit approach to health coverage. While there is some evidence of movement by smaller employers to defined-contribution health benefits, the practical barriers to broader adoption are sobering.[21] Removing individuals from group coverage throws them into an expensive and volatile market for individual coverage. This could increase the cost to employees of achieving the same package of benefits by as much as 30 to 40 percent. That is the typical difference between the premiums offered to large groups and those offered to individuals, without the large group's clout and purchasing power.

If all the employer does is give employees a lump sum salary increase equal to what they were previously spending on health insurance premiums, employees get a most unwelcome increase in their taxable income. Employers could continue deducting the amount as a salary expense, but the benefit would no longer be tax free, as health benefits are, to employees. This would take an additional 20 to 40 percent bite out of the health benefits apple. Between the loss of group rates and the taxation, a very significant fraction of the economic value of the health benefit to the employee disappears.

There are ways around both of these problems. Employers that incorporate defined-contribution health coverage into a "cafeteria style" benefits plan can take advantage of an existing federal law facilitating movement of benefit dollars between types of benefit (health insurance, vacation, retirement, etc.). The federal tax law could be further amended to provide that defined contributions by the employer for health coverage outside of a cafeteria plan could remain tax free to employees.

Mechanisms can also be found to pool the purchasing power of employees so that they would not have to enter the health insurance market individually through buyer's clubs or multiple-employer purchasing pools. Indeed, Internet-based health insurance purchasing exchanges, employing the technologies discussed above, could play a crucial role in preserving employee purchasing power in health insurance markets. Congressional advocates have referred to these pooling mechanisms as "health marts."

Nevertheless, employer health contributions in future years are unlikely to keep pace with the rise in premiums, forcing employees under a defined-contribution approach to contribute more of their own funds to pay for coverage. Healthcare use will change as this happens, but whether these savings will be enough to offset potentially large cost increases borne by the employee remains to be seen.

THE WOLF BY THE EARS

Because they remain at risk for the health costs of more than 130 million Americans, finding new ways of controlling health costs is an urgent task for health plans. Private health insurers have been systematically stripped of the tools they have used in the past to control medical costs. Those tools included demanding discounts from providers in exchange for (allegedly) bringing them new business, excluding or restricting access to specialists, externally reviewing and challenging the medical necessity of procedures, and simply clogging the claims payment pipeline with bureaucratic processes.

Private health insurance premiums have resumed rising at double-digit rates as of this writing, after almost a decade of relative calm. Simply increasing prices, as health plans tend to do when they are in economic trouble, may provide them a short-term infusion of cash. But rate increases do nothing to justify the health plan's removal of between 10 and 20 percent of the premium before actually paying the hospital and doctors.

For better or worse, private health plans remain responsible to employers for containing health costs. To paraphrase Jefferson's comment about the United States and slavery at the turn of the nineteenth century, private health insurers "have the wolf by the ears." Unless they can discover new leverage points for containing health costs and actually contribute to improving the quality of care, they will be eaten alive by the health cost wolf.

The most important emerging leverage point is likely to be the consumer's household budget. It makes powerful intuitive sense that individuals will spend their own money more carefully than they will spend the employer's money. It is clear that without a greater economic stake in conservative health use by consumers, health costs will not come under control.

CONSUMERS WILL PAY MORE FOR THEIR CHOICES

Despite their perception of steadily rising personal contributions, the consumer's share of national health expenditures has fallen steadily over the past 40 years (Figure 6.1). Notably, it fell even during the period of the managed care revolution (the 1980s and 1990s), because employers used reduced cost sharing as a way of encouraging people to enroll in health plans.

Another way of viewing this is that economic risk steadily shifted toward the employer and private health insurance during the managed care explosion, and away from consumers. Moreover, the structure of that cost sharing—a nominal copayment of the insurance premium, variable amounts of "first dollar" deductibles for various forms of healthcare use (focused primarily on the hospitalization), and a maximum annual cap on the consumer's cost exposure—had not changed materially in 30 years.

Health plans are already experimenting with the use of economic incentives as a way of encouraging consumers to use less expensive providers of service by varying the cost share depending on the "tier" of hospital they visit. People who use their community hospitals for most of their care will pay less out of pocket than people who rely entirely on expensive academic health centers for all their care. So far, the anecdotal evidence suggests that consumers are willing to pay more out of pocket to use expensive institutions and that the incentives have not encouraged much switching.

Health plans have had some success containing pharmacy expense through so-called "three-tier" pharmacy coverage. Under three-tier coverage, the managed care plan or the pharmacy benefits manager negotiates a list of approved drugs for which subscribers

Figure 6.1: Consumers' Out-of-Pocket Spending as Share of Total Health Costs

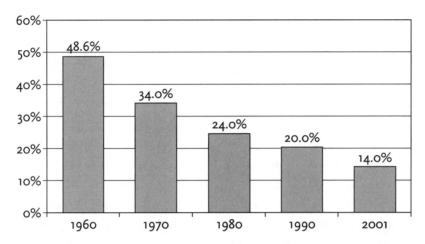

Source: U.S. Centers for Medicaid & Medicare Services, National Health Expenditure Projections, 2002.

are eligible and obtains discounts from drug companies for placing their drugs on the list, which is called a formulary.

Under this plan, consumers who use generic drugs on the formulary have nominal or no cost share. Consumers who use approved "branded drugs" on the formulary pay a modest cost share. Consumers who want to use a branded drug not on the formulary may pay as much as half of the cost out of pocket. For example, the average tier 1 copayment is $7.17, whereas the tier 2 copayment is $14.14 and the tier 3 copayment can be as high as $27.35.[22]

Although some questions still linger about how lasting the effects of these incentives will be, health plans that used triple-tier pharmacy coverage were able to cut the rate of escalation of their prescription drug expenses in half compared to open-ended plans. Not surprisingly, measures to outlaw the three-tier approach were slipped into patient-protection legislation in many states by aggressive pharmaceutical company lobbying.

IMPLICATIONS FOR HOSPITALS AND PHYSICIANS

The digitized, consumer-centric model of health insurance has numerous implications for hospitals and physicians. Increased transparency of clinical results and cost will mean that high cost and high-risk hospitals and physicians could lose market share as consumers move to safer or higher-value alternatives. This risk embodies powerful reasons for hospitals and physicians to collaborate in improving patient safety, as well as to increase efficiency and customer service.

Increased cost sharing will probably increase bad debts for providers of all types and friction with patients in collecting those debts. Hospitals and physicians will become increasingly visible as a source of health cost increases as the veil of third-party insurance is partially stripped away. (It will probably also catalyze some type of political reaction against health providers, particularly if the burden of cost sharing is, as it presently seems to be, not equitably distributed by income class.)

The good news, however, is that digitizing health plan operations could also help reduce the lag in payment that presently afflicts the paper-clogged healthcare payment system. Interactive claims management between hospitals, doctors, and health plans could lead to instantaneous electronic payment for health services, markedly reducing not only accounts receivable, but also clerical expense on both ends of the transaction. Hospitals and physicians must be prepared to digitize their back offices and connect their claims systems to health insurers via the Internet.

As suggested earlier, nurses and hospital personnel presently wrestling the paperwork monster of antiquated healthcare payment schemes could be reassigned to supporting continuity of care and communication with patients. Thus, consumer-centric health insurance, enabled by modern IT, is a two-headed coin, simultaneously restructuring relationships and simplifying transactions in healthcare services and payment.

CAN HEALTH INSURANCE BECOME A
CONSUMER-DRIVEN BUSINESS?

Implementing change is the soft underbelly of any health enterprise. Health plans have been strangled by the sheer magnitude of their back-office problems. Just as with hospitals, health plans must have modern enterprise information systems before they can fix the customer service problems that have plagued them.

Health plans certainly have as much incentive to change their business model as any actor in the healthcare system. If physicians face the crippling inability to take collective action and hospitals struggle with an anarchic clash of professional interests and cultures, then health plans will struggle with a legacy of paternalism and insensitivity to the needs of the consumer and family.

Among the health plans, perhaps the most aggressive IT innovator has been Humana. Humana not only has invested $1 billion in the last four years to renovate and computerize its back office, but it has also invested in a suite of consumer applications to bring "consumer directed" health plan options to its members. Blending web-enabled health plan customization with sharp increases in cost sharing for hospital services, Humana was able to reduce its own employees' health benefits cost escalation from 19 percent per year to under 5 percent in the first two years of its new plan.[23] If Humana's early results are any indication, IT-enabled, consumer-centric health insurance may be good business for health plans, as well as welcome news to employers and consumers frightened by explosive health cost increases.

Delivering promised improvements in service is the true test of good intentions by health plans. If, as it is said in architecture, God is in the details, in e-commerce, God is in the back end. Administrative systems in health plans need to be completely renovated and digitized for any of the promising Internet tools discussed above to make any difference.

The emergence of the Internet has given health plans a potential lifeline. Properly executed, Internet applications can help health plans rebuild their relationships with hospitals and physicians by reducing or eliminating paperwork and bureaucratic interference with medical practice. IT can also give them the leverage needed to help their subscribers make more sensible healthcare decisions.

Information technology enabled by the Internet can, again if properly executed, bring tangible benefits to consumers that will help them make constructive use of the choice they have demanded. In addition, information systems strategies can help health plans offset a significant percentage of the present cost rise with improved productivity and efficiency and more responsible consumer choices.

Connectivity makes all organizations more transparent and accountable to customers. Health plans that embrace the need for openness and responsiveness will find their position in the health system strengthened in future years. The health plans that succeed in the digital transformation will not only survive, but also prosper.

NOTES

1. Taylor, H., and R. Leitman, eds. 2001. "Consumer Backlash Against Managed Care and Pharmaceutical Industries—Bottomed Out or In Remission." *Harris Interactive* 1 (17): 1–4.

2. Taylor, H., and R. Leitman, eds. 2001. "The Managed Care Paradox: Many Dislike Managed Care, Yet They Like Their Own Health Plans." *Harris Interactive* 1 (6): 1–5.

3. Lord, J. 2001. Humana Corporation. Personal communication, May.

4. Briggs, B. 2000. "Electronic Claims Growth Plods Ahead." *Health Data Management* 8 (9): 70–74.

5. Faulkner and Gray. 2000. *Health Data Directory, 2000 Edition*. New York: Faulkner and Gray.

6. Malcolm, C. 2000. Computer Sciences Corporation. Personal communication, May.

7. Dorenfest, S. 2000. "The Decade of the 90s." *Healthcare Informatics* 17 (8): 64–67.

8. Downes, L., and C. Mui. 1998. *Unleashing the Killer App: Digital Strategies for Market Dominance*. Boston: Harvard Business School Press.

9. Lathrop, J. P., G. Ahlquist, and D. G. Knott. 2000. "Healthcare's New Electronic Marketplace." *Strategy+Business,* 2nd Quarter, 36.

10. Kongstvedt, P., and H. Shaman. 2000. *Managed Care Measures: Result of the 1999 Benchmarking Study.* Washington, DC: Ernst & Young.

11. Ibid. Faulkner and Gray.

12. Ibid. Malcolm, C.

13. Ibid. Kongstvedt, P., and H. Shaman.

14. Center for Studying Health System Change. 2002. "Community Tracking Study: Physician Survey." [Online information; retrieved 12/30/02.] http://www.hschange .com/index.cgi?data=04.

15. Wennberg, J. E., and M. M. Cooper, eds. 1999. "The Quality of Medical Care in the United States: A Report on the Medicare Program." *The Dartmouth Atlas of Healthcare in the United States.* Chicago: American Hospital Publishing.

16. Tieman, J. 2002. "HHS Backs Industry's Quality Plan." *Modern Healthcare.* [Online information; retrieved 1/6/03.] http://www.modernhealthcare .com/news.cms?newsId=375.

17. Millenson, M. 1997. *Demanding Medical Excellence: Doctors and Accountability in the Information Age.* Chicago: University of Chicago Press.

18. Gustafson, D. H., R. Hawkins, E. Boberg, S. Pingree, R. E. Serlin, F. Graziano, and C. L. Chan. 1999. "Impact of Patient-centered Computer-based Health Information/Support System (CHESS)." *American Journal of Preventive Medicine* 16 (1): 1–9.

19. Ibid. Wennberg, J., and M. Cooper.

20. Goldsmith, J. C. 2000. "The Internet and Managed Care: A New Wave of Innovation." *Health Affairs* 19 (6): 42–56.

21. Ibid. Kongstvedt, P., and H. Shaman.

22. Pharmacy Benefit Management Institute. 2001. Report for Takeda Pharmaceuticals and Eli Lilly and Company, October.

23. Ibid. Lord, J.

CHAPTER 7

Health Policy Issues Raised by Information Technology

THE PROFOUND CHANGES in business policy and relationships in medicine brought about by information technology inevitably take on a political dimension. How government responds to these political pressures and how it structures payment for health services under the Medicare and Medicaid programs will affect both the speed and universality of the changes discussed in this book. The central issues policymakers must address are the following:

1. Protecting medical privacy
2. Standardizing clinical software
3. Changing healthcare payment methodology

Each of these issues will be discussed below.

PROTECTING MEDICAL PRIVACY

Outside of the family, nothing rivals the intimacy of the physician-patient relationship in American society. Personal health information is the most intimate documentary information that exists in the

U.S. economy. Someone with access to this information knows a person's most carefully guarded secrets—personal medical and psychiatric history, sexual orientation and history, lifestyles and their risks, drug history, and a lot of things about relationships with others. Insurers who see the totality of someone's healthcare use can use that information to estimate how good or bad an insurance risk he or she may be in the future and decide not only if they wish to provide coverage, but also how much to charge for it.

That patients disclose this information to physicians is vital to ensuring optimal care. Physicians require it because making intelligent treatment decisions is based on understanding medical and personal history and the impact of those decisions on health. Anonymous medicine is expensive and dangerous medicine. If physicians cannot be trusted with intimate personal knowledge, the opportunity for injury or death escalates alarmingly.

Yet this intimate doctor-patient relationship is really a three-way relationship, in which only two of the parties are physically present. Despite its intimacy, medical information is also among the most widely distributed and poorly protected personal information in our society. Thanks to federal legislation passed in the wake of the highly publicized Congressional hearings of Supreme Court Justice Clarence Thomas, video rental records were actually safer from disclosure than a patient's medical records. Consumers' personal health information is an open book lying out on the desk.

How can this be? The main reason is that health costs have grown to the point that they are no longer an affordable personal responsibility. As a direct consequence, third parties, typically employers and the health insurers they hire to manage their health costs, demand access to this information. With the growth in managed care, health plans use personal health information to establish whether the healthcare they pay for is necessary and appropriate.

Because insurers and employers have an economic incentive to minimize their outlays, their interest in obtaining personal medical information has acquired a pungent adversarial odor. Employers with access to employees' health history may decide they no longer wish to employ someone or invest in training or promoting that person into a leadership position to avoid being responsible for their medical costs.

When someone sees a physician or visits a hospital, he or she is typically required to sign a release that authorizes the provider to release whatever information the health insurer may require to review the medical claim arising from the visit. The result is a legal authorization for the physician to breach medical confidentiality in order to get paid. Study a medical information release the next time you are asked to sign one. You will be amazed at how open ended it is.

The information patients authorize physicians to release is not only compared to the health plan's contract to ensure that the service is covered by the health plan. It is also compared to the information provided about the employee's medical history when he or she enrolled in the health plan.

The purpose of this review is to determine if the condition for which the patient is being treated predates enrollment in the health plan. If it does, but the employee did not disclose that precondition, the plan can not only refuse to pay the claim, but it may also move to invalidate coverage on the grounds that the employee misrepresented his or her health status. Employees may even be sued for fraud if the health plan can prove that they willfully withheld information and lied when attesting to the completeness of their health history.

Because people frequently switch health plans, an individual health plan may not have a complete picture of their medical history and claims experience. As a consequence, health insurers have created medical information clearinghouses, which aggregate medical information from diverse sources. Insurers routinely draw on this source of information to obtain additional information about consumers to determine if there is a reason to avoid paying their medical claims.

The health information in these bureaus is technically available only to health insurers. In practice, however, it is available on demand to law enforcement agencies, which can obtain access to it merely by asking for it. They do not even require a court-issued search warrant; they can just send a letter and obtain health information without the knowledge or consent of the person involved.

Also, like virtually every other computerized database, medical information is accessible to computer hackers who "break and enter" the provider, insurer, or clearinghouse database. When they do, at least until recently, they face minimal penalties. In 2000, a hacker broke into the clinical information system at the University of Washington's principal teaching hospital and obtained extensive personal health histories on a number of patients. His alleged purpose was to demonstrate how insecure this information was and how easily it could be obtained.

How Concerns About Medical Privacy Change Our Behavior

Many consumers do not trust the handling of their personal health information. According to a poll commissioned by the California HealthCare Foundation in 1999, one in five Americans believes that a healthcare provider, health plan, government agency, or employer has improperly disclosed personal health information.[1] Half of this group believed it resulted in personal embarrassment or harm. According to an earlier Harris poll, 27 percent of the public believed that their personal health information had been improperly disclosed, and one-third of this group felt that they had been harmed or embarrassed by the disclosure.[2]

To protect their privacy, consumers often compromise their own health by avoiding care for sensitive medical problems. Alternatively, they may elect to pay for such care out of pocket, even though services are covered by their plans, to avoid creating a record of the problem for which they are being treated. One in six Americans in the California HealthCare Foundation survey said they did something out of the ordinary to keep personal medical information confidential, including providing inaccurate or incomplete information to their doctors, doctor-hopping to avoid a consolidated record, or other strategies. Some 11 percent of those surveyed by the Harris poll chose not to file claims on health services they did not want in their medical records, and 7 percent had chosen not to seek care because they did not want to harm their "job prospects or other life opportunities."

The Privacy Unconcerned

Not everyone feels this way. Alan Westin, a professor of law at Columbia University who has studied consumer attitudes toward privacy for many years, says, "The average person today is engaged in a level of self-disclosure that is truly unparalleled in the history of Western civilization."[3] A surprising amount of this self-disclosure is entirely voluntary.

Scott MacNealy, CEO of Sun Microsystems, once counseled, "You have zero privacy anyway. Get over it." A significant, although shrinking, number of Americans are blissfully unaware of how little privacy they have. Westin calls these people the "privacy unconcerned." Until recently, they comprised about 20 percent of the population. Westin believes this number has shrunk by half with the recent wave of publicity about privacy risks, particularly on the Internet.[4]

Privacy Fundamentalists

Another roughly 25 percent are what Westin calls "privacy fundamentalists," whose personal experiences have led them to be profoundly suspicious and mistrustful of sharing personal information. Fundamentalists not only alter their behavior to avoid disclosing personal information via computer systems and the Internet, but they are also a formidable force in shaping public opinion about public policy protections for privacy, in the health sphere and elsewhere.

Privacy Pragmatists

In the middle, constituting well more than half the population, are what Westin calls "privacy pragmatists," people who believe that the benefits they derive from using the Internet and other information tools justify some sacrifice of personal privacy. Most of us accept some of these tradeoffs, even if we may not fully understand the terms of trade.

Included in the pragmatist category are people who are seduced into providing detailed personal profiles of their spending habits, values, and attitudes in exchange for free Internet access or other goodies. How many so-called pragmatists actually evaluate the terms of trade respecting their privacy is an open and interesting research question. For many, what Westin calls "pragmatism" may stem from being uninformed at a deeper level about the extent of privacy risk.

How I Became a Privacy Fundamentalist

Health information is special, and people are especially sensitive to how it is used. According to Westin, the number of people who are fundamentalists about health information is 45 percent of the population.[5] They have good reasons to be sensitive, and I learned some of them firsthand.

In my wildest dreams, I never imagined that, little more than two years after finishing my graduate education at the University of Chicago, I would be returning there as a medical school administrator. My graduate student career at Chicago's superb Social Sciences Division was extraordinarily stimulating. I left in a hurry in the summer of 1973, with the ink barely dry on my doctorate, to pursue a career in public policy in the State of Illinois Governor's Office.

In the fall of 1975, however, an opportunity arose to return as an assistant to a dynamic new dean of the University of Chicago's Pritzker School of Medicine. We got along well, and I was offered the position despite my lack of experience with health administration or biomedical science. The position required a preemployment physical in the university's employee and student health service.

I reported for my physical late on a Friday afternoon. A state plane was waiting at Meigs Field to return some colleagues and me, after my exam, to Springfield for an urgent late night meeting with the governor and his staff regarding our dispute with Mayor Richard J. Daley (father of today's Mayor Richard M. Daley) over funding the Chicago Board of Education. This dispute was front-page news in Chicago, and our meetings were fraught with tremendous stress as they were recorded by television cameras and as reporters shouted questions.

The medical resident in employee health who performed my physical was extraordinarily meticulous and detailed in his examination. It seemed endless, and despite an explanation of the circumstances and gentle prodding on my part, he refused to shorten the exam. I eventually made my airplane and returned to Springfield.

When I returned to my office, the dean's secretary had contacted me to let me know that the dean wished to discuss my mental health history prior to finalizing my appointment to his staff. "What mental health history?" I remember asking. My "mental health" history consisted of a note in my student health medical record regarding my request for sleeping pills needed during the time that I was writing my dissertation (after writing for 18 hours a day, it was sometimes very difficult to turn off the engine and get to sleep).

This request triggered a routine note to my chart referring me to student mental health for follow-up counseling, apparently a standard operating practice. I had no idea this note was even part of my medical record, because no one actually spoke with me about the referral. I was focusing like a laser beam on finishing my dissertation and getting a good job, both of which I did.

My urgent desire to finish my preemployment physical and return to Springfield for my meeting led the resident to diagnose me with an "anxiety" disorder. The governor did get really frosty with people who were late for meetings, so I guess I might have seemed anxious to someone who didn't know the circumstances. However, I know I also rubbed the resident (who was exactly my age and remarkably pompous and officious for a 26 year old) the wrong way. I had unwittingly challenged his authority by urging him to finish his work.

The resident rewarded me for my presumptuousness by contacting the head of the student health service about my "mental health" problem, who in turn contacted the dean and suggested that I might be a "high risk" hire. All this resulted in an unwelcome inquiry into the state of my mental health with my new employer. The dean understood the circumstances and hired me anyway. Thus began my career in health services.

The story does not end there, however. Two years later, a member of my family had a medical problem that required hospital attention. When we went to settle the bill with our health insurer, we received a denial on the grounds that I, not my family member, had concealed a "pre-existing condition" (my "mental health history") from the insurer when I enrolled in the plan. Therefore, our health insurance contract, and any claim we may have to benefits for anyone in my family, was invalid. There ensued numerous angry volleys of correspondence before the insurer relented and paid our family's claim.

This incident both enraged and frightened me. I felt violated. I realized that even seemingly incidental contact with the health system could leave a trail that persisted for years afterward, potentially compromising my and my family's health insurance status. The incident in employee health was like cadmium in my well water, permanent and unwelcome. My trust in the guardians of my medical secrets was permanently diminished. The question of how the information I provide my physicians could be used always follows me into the exam room or physician's office.

What disturbed me most about the incident was my total lack of recourse. I could do precisely nothing about the inaccurate entries in my record, because I had no right even to see my medical record, let alone to amend it. Nor could I obtain a copy of the report filed with the medical information bureau on the basis of which my claim was challenged. The laws have since changed, but the bureaucratic inertia and sensibility that produced my problem have not.

Electronic Health Information

Three technological forces—the digitization of health information, the revolution in connectivity represented by the Internet, and the impending arrival of genetic information in the electronic patient record—will raise the saliency of medical privacy concerns to a whole new level.

To an unappreciated extent, the fact that most medical records were in paper form actually protected privacy. Paper charts can be "sampled" by prying eyes, but only if the snoopy person can find them to examine. While they can be copied or stolen, medical records are bulky and cumbersome. The larger they are, the more difficult they are to duplicate. Some hospital medical records are large enough to use for doorstops or weapons (an older person's medical record has an impressive throw weight). They can also be destroyed, which may be bad for patient care, but good for privacy.

Digitization turns medical information from a solid block in a single place into a kind of aerosol spray. Thanks to Internet connectivity, a person's most intimate medical secrets have become, to a degree unprecedented in human experience, mobile and portable. Once digitized and unleashed into electronic networks, medical information can literally turn up anywhere and will move through broadband networks like quicksilver.

Consumers have already learned with e-mail how easy it is to reconstruct electronic communications. One may have the comforting illusion when deleting an e-mail from a personal computer that it is gone, but it continues to reside on multiple servers. It is remarkably easy both for authorities and for hackers to retrieve electronic communications from multiple storage places in both corporate and regional electronic networks.

Electronic communications are reliably insecure. It is not for nothing that privacy experts advise that one should put nothing in an e-mail that one is uncomfortable writing on a postcard. No sane person would put his or her medical secrets on a postcard.

The benefits of easy movement of clinical information in the health system are obvious. Uncertainty is the enemy of effective medical treatment. Potential patients need not be strangers to any health provider they choose to use if connectivity can deliver their electronic medical record to the point of care. The ability to project accurate information about a patient's health to the point of care can reduce the uncertainty about who they are, what is wrong with them, and how to help them, lowering the risk of a bad outcome.

The impending demand for genetic information in the medical record (for reasons discussed in Chapter 2) raises the ante in any discussion of medical privacy policy. As was suggested above, the electronic patient record (or more accurately, the intelligent clinical information system which uses that record) is the emerging thread of continuity between consumers/patients and the health system. Genetic information will be a vital component of that record necessary to avoid medication errors and to focus and direct treatment of an individual's disease. Patients will not contribute their genetic information to a patient record that they do not trust as secure and privacy protected. Thus, privacy concerns could hamper the adoption of powerful genetic tools to improve patient care.

The technological challenges associated with greater levels of security and privacy of medical records are not massive. Sophisticated encryption technology and password systems to control access to electronic files are routinely used in other businesses. Virtual private networks (VPNs) can electronically segregate communications channels among providers, and between providers and health insurers, from broader Internet traffic. VPNs can provide a further level of security in communicating patient records across large distances. Taken together and administered thoughtfully, these tools can make the electronic record far more secure than the paper records they replaced. However, to ensure that these tools are used properly, there must not only be industry consensus on procedures and standards regarding access and a legal framework to enforce restrictions, but there must also be a sense of urgency about using the available tools to secure vital health knowledge.

STANDARDIZING CLINICAL SOFTWARE

In 1996, in the wake of the failure of health reform, Congress passed a deceptively influential piece of legislation called the Health Insurance Portability and Accountability Act (HIPAA). The principal goal of HIPAA (sometimes referred to as the Kassebaum-Kennedy Act) was to make it easier for those who changed jobs or lost their job to retain their health benefits and to make benefits more portable from employer to employer.

Despite its baffling title and seemingly modest goal, HIPAA was the most important piece of healthcare legislation passed by Congress since the enactment of Medicare in 1965 because it anticipated expanded electronic commerce in healthcare. It assumed that transactions between consumers, health insurers, and providers would eventually be in electronic form (although not, given when the law was drafted, through the Internet).

As discussed earlier, the health system is tremendously fragmented among health plans, among healthcare providers, and between the two factions. To make electronic commerce in medicine easier, HIPAA created federal standards for formatting trans-actions and for coding both clinical and financial information to be transmitted electronically. These standards apply to all healthcare transactions, not merely those of the federal Medicare program. HIPAA also imposed new—and costly—standards for protection of the privacy and security of personal health information.

There was precedent for federal standard setting in electronic commerce. Federal rules standardized electronic transactions in banking, creating universal coding and routing conventions that permit wire transfers between banks (the machine-readable codes on the bottom of checks). However, health payment transactions are logarithmically more complex than banking transactions.

HIPAA's "administrative simplification" provisions will make it much easier for health plans to communicate with consumers, physicians, and hospitals because they will all be speaking, in effect, the same language. Administrative simplification will eventually save billions of dollars in reduced clerical costs and delays in payment. It will do this by making it easier to substitute instantaneous electronic communication for paper and telephone communication.[6]

Issues Triggered by HIPAA

HIPAA did something far more important than merely standardizing electronic commerce inside the health system. It set federal standards governing the privacy and security of personal medical information. It required providers, health insurers, and their business partners to establish stringent privacy protections for personal health information. The law also required healthcare providers to use encryption technology to protect any confidential medical information transmitted electronically. The following sections discuss issues that triggered reactions to the legislation from various players involved.

Disclosure of Information

HIPAA requires hospitals, doctors, pharmacies, and others to develop policies to control who gets access to personal health information and for what reasons and to track the use of medical records to ensure that these policies are enforced. HIPAA requires all providers to obtain written consent for any use of personal information for normal "treatment, payment and healthcare operations" (provisions fundamentally weakened by the enabling regulations issued by the Department of Health and Human Services [HHS] in mid-2002). HIPAA also federally established consumers' right to see and correct errors in their medical record.

Furthermore, the law required specific written authorization by consumers for use of their personal health information for any purpose other than "treatment, payment or routine healthcare operations." Institutions or individuals that knowingly violate a consumer's right to medical privacy may be punished with fines and imprisonment. These regulations were fully implemented in spring 2003.

Cost to Hospitals and Providers

Despite the health industry spending billions in campaign contributions and lobbying expenses to protect their interests, HIPAA passed under the health industry's radar. The cost implications were not fully understood until almost three years after the legislation was passed. It was only when draft regulations to implement the legislation began trickling out of HHS that providers and insurers glimpsed the magnitude of the cost challenge they face in complying with HIPAA's provisions.

Lobbying organizations representing hospitals and health insurers belatedly but vigorously resisted HIPAA's privacy regulations. The health system had some justification for objecting. No federal funds were appropriated to help with the expensive information systems conversions required by HIPAA. Furthermore, Medicare outlays for services to the elderly had not risen in the four years from 1997 to 2000, despite rising wages, expensive new drugs and technology, and increasing numbers of elderly people.

HIPAA's mandates were galling to hard-pressed hospitals, doctors, and health plans because the government was simultaneously freezing or cutting payment to them and requiring major capital expenses to comply with the new law. When the Bush administration came to power, intense political pressure was brought to bear by health industry lobbyists on the new regime to delay or water down HIPAA's regulations to mitigate their cost impact.

Universal Patient Identification

Interestingly and not surprisingly, civil liberties groups objected strenuously to the HIPAA requirement that a universal patient identifier be created. This personal identifier would be attached to every person's medical records, replacing the ubiquitous and inappropriately used social security number. It would make Enterprise Master Patient Index (EMPI) software, which is used to cross-reference multiple patient records in hospitals, unnecessary.

This single health identifier would enable all of a person's medical records from different providers to be aggregated more easily into a single record. Civil libertarians lacked confidence in the privacy and confidentiality provisions in the law and believed that the easier it is to aggregate health information, the easier it is for employers or insurers to abuse employees' rights.

The Internet Development Post-HIPAA

HIPAA was enacted on the cusp of the Internet boom and did not fully foresee the emergence of application service providers (ASPs), consumer web sites, and Internet-based electronic medical connectivity. As Cunningham and others have pointed out, HIPAA has complicated federal policy toward e-health because it was based on a pre-Internet model of health data interchange. Cunningham put it well in a late-2000 analysis: "HIPAA's IT provisions are now cast in a doubly problematic light, simultaneously behind the times and crowding the road ahead with mandates."[7]

In the waning days of the Clinton administration, HHS issued regulations extending HIPAA privacy and security protections to nonelectronic (e.g., oral and written) patient information as well, probably broadening federal oversight beyond the scope intended by Congress. The HIPAA regulations also extended the protections to business partners in an attempt to advance the regulatory protections to new Internet actors such as Internet service providers (ISPs) and ASPs whose emerging roles were not anticipated by HIPAA's drafters.

Why HIPAA Did Not Go Far Enough

In the discussion of genetic prediction, I suggested that the health system would be acquiring in the next few years the capacity to glimpse into our personal health destinies through genetic diagnosis. Genetic testing will exquisitely personalize medical treatment and identify our vulnerability to various treatment options. Eventually, genetic prediction will permit an increasingly fine-grained assessment of inherited disease risk and enable an entirely new mission of the health system—predicting and managing disease risk in advance of illness.[8]

However, these very same tools could enable health insurers or employers to identify with far greater precision the high-risk, and potentially high-cost, employees in their insurance pools, based on their genetic predisposition to expensive diseases. Without stringent protections, this information could be used to deny consumers insurance coverage and compromise their access to care. After all, in a genetic world, most major illness will stem from a "pre-existing condition," since they will be determined to flow, albeit in a mysterious way, from specific, identifiable genetic abnormalities.

Insurers have historically attempted to limit their exposure to conditions that predate an employee's entry into their insurance risk pool. They know that consumers make very intelligent short-run decisions to obtain coverage for anticipated medical conditions. People anticipating having a baby or an elective surgical procedure will often opt for higher levels of coverage (and lower levels of personal cost exposure) for those conditions by changing health plans.

Health plans that do not guard against this shifting risk are hammered with what, in insurance jargon, is known as "adverse selection." Health insurance costs are always estimated as group averages. The bigger the group, the more confident the actuarial forecast of future health expenses will be. A few hundred-thousand-dollar medical "incidents" (known in the health insurance industry as "shock claims") will blow the economic cost of covering a group sky high, resulting in losses for the risk-bearing entity (either the employer or the insurer).

Avoiding these losses is a major reason why health insurers want to continue to have unfettered access to employees' medical secrets and unlimited discretion in deciding what they will cover. Unless preexisting conditions clauses are outlawed and access to genetic information on disease risk is restricted, the advent of genetic prediction will enable insurers to avoid future health costs by excluding those with potentially expensive forms of genetic disease risk.

HIPAA contained restrictions on the use by health plans of family history information (which is a proxy for genetic information) for enrolling Medicare patients in health plans. The health insurance industry is waging a quiet struggle to preserve its options in the face of new genetic predictive tools. Consumers must become aware of this still largely hidden struggle, and weigh into the public debate over the appropriate use of genetic information.

Standardization

The fact that HIPAA did not foresee the explosion of connectivity that would sweep the health system is not the only reason for Congress to revisit health information policy. The reality is that attempts to use the powerful new tools discussed in this book in the current fragmented information systems and the vast sprawl of competing health providers could result in huge waste and inefficiency.

No one clinical software vendor dominates its space in the way Microsoft dominates software for personal computers. Moreover, the struggle for market share by these vendors does not seem likely to produce a "market" solution to standard clinical information system formats any time soon. Proceeding on the current course could easily result in expenditures by hospitals alone of more than $100 billion to digitize clinical record systems that do not communicate from hospital to hospital or from hospitals to physicians because the software is incompatible and does not interoperate.

Clinical Software

HIPAA did not address these problems because they were not foreseeable when the law was enacted. To speed adoption of new clinical IT, the federal government should require that providers convert their paper records into electronic form to qualify for Medicare payment. Once this electronic record is in place, the federal government should require that hospitals install computerized physician order entry systems with clinical decision support to enable IT systems to evaluate and strengthen physicians' ordering practices to ensure safety.

To be sure that records are comparable from hospital to hospital, the federal government should specify minimum technical standards for clinical information systems: common coding schemes and record structure, controlled medical vocabulary, and a common clinical messaging format that all vendors would be required to use. Again, this can be enforced by making Medicare payment contingent on use of systems that comply with the standards.

This degree of standardization would not eliminate competition in the clinical software industry. Vendors would be free to compete, as they do today, not only on price, but ease and speed of installation, latency (speed of system response), stability and reliability, user friendliness, and most importantly, depth and sophistication of "knowledgeware"—clinical decision support. Vendors have many opportunities to differentiate their offerings while conforming to a set of minimal technical standards.

Medical Error Reporting

Because physician order information would be entered in a standard format and the resulting clinical outcomes recorded in a standard format, it would be easy for institutions to track (and therefore to report and disclose publicly) the level of medication errors and other medical errors in healthcare institutions of all types on a uniform basis. They could be reported "blinded" as to practitioner to protect them from malpractice litigation. It is likely that accrediting bodies such as the Joint Commission of Accreditation of Healthcare Organizations will require the use of clinical software to monitor and evaluate care patterns as a condition of hospitals obtaining accreditation.

Having specified a minimal clinical information infrastructure for a safer health system, federal law should provide a malpractice "safe harbor" for institutions and practitioners who use these tools, including clinical outcome guidelines. There is precedent here, in the decision by malpractice insurers to rate those anesthesiologists who used pulse oximetry to monitor patient conditions in surgery as safer and eligible for lower rates. Safer patients will mean fewer malpractice actions and lower malpractice rates.

The federal government should also require that (1) all providers submit their claims electronically via the Internet to Medicare in an interactive format that permits the claims to be evaluated and paid electronically as well and (2) Medicare, through its intermediaries, pay within a certain short period of time upon submittal of a clean claim. More than 85 percent of all Medicare claims are presently filed in electronic form, but much of this is in tape format, which is not fully interactive. The ability to verify coverage and obtain payment quickly, as well as to resolve Medicare billing problems in real time, rather than through paper and telephone interactions, will save the federal government and providers a small fortune in reduced clerical expenses.

Furthermore, the federal government should also move beyond the Administrative Simplification provisions of HIPAA to specify that health insurers require a common set of claims justifications or documentation to evaluate a claim for payment. HIPAA standardizes the format for claims attachments, but it does not sufficiently narrow the diverse data requests of different health insurers to actually reduce provider billing costs. The lack of standardization of health plans' data requirements is a major lingering source of unnecessary administrative expense for healthcare providers.

Funding the Standardization Process

Unlike HIPAA, new federal legislation should recognize that the cost of these mandates may exceed the ability of many health providers. Thousands of small hospitals and practitioners will not have the cash, credit, or technical staff to make the transition from paper to electronic charts and billing systems. They will need federal assistance, perhaps in the form of a Hill-Burton-type program. Hill-Burton provided federal matching funds to hospital construction in the decades immediately following World War II in response to a perceived shortage of hospital beds. An alternative would be to create an annex to Medicare hospital and physician payments, perhaps graded to serving underserved populations, to provide additional cash flow to cover IT acquisition costs.

Wealthy institutions should perhaps receive some token federal assistance to underscore the timeliness of needed information system renovations. But it is not sensible to substitute tax dollars for private dollars that would voluntarily have been spent digitizing hospitals' clinical and operating systems.

Other Challenges and Considerations

Earlier, it was argued that hospitals and physicians ought not to maintain the present balkanized medical information structure, with separate and nonlinkable medical records in the hospital and the physician's office. Even where the climate of collaboration between hospitals and physicians would permit a common record system to emerge, present federal laws raise barriers. Hospitals that provided connection by physicians to a clinical record system could be construed as violating federal fraud and abuse regulations, which forbid hospitals from offering services or payment to physicians for using their facilities (the modern variant of an ancient and ethically indefensible practice known as "fee splitting").

Moreover, for the 85 percent of all hospitals that are presently not-for-profit, federal and state tax laws forbid them from providing physicians anything of value. If inurement provisions did not exist, many not-for-profit institutions would function as mere front organizations for profit-making enterprises, funneling tax-free dollars into individuals' and businesses' pockets.

However, changes in federal law could work to minimize these risks in the public benefit. If clinical information systems by different vendors all used common formats, medical vocabularies, and coding schemes, no provider could achieve market leverage by "locking in" physicians to using their proprietary medical records system, and the fraud and abuse risk could be alleviated. On the not-for-profit issue, one could reasonably argue for exempting clinical information systems from inurement provisions on the grounds of markedly improved patient safety resulting from the free flow of clinical information among all the diverse actors in medicine.

I strongly believe in market solutions to economic problems. Moreover, an ethos of personal responsibility for health and health costs is vital to containing future health cost increases. However, the present policy climate in clinical information, on both the vendor and provider sides, approaches anarchy. Tens of thousand of lives are needlessly lost every year because of inadequate or poorly coordinated care. Creating the infrastructure and decision support to improve standards of care is a legitimate job for government.[9]

HEALTHCARE PAYMENT METHODOLOGY

A Subscription Model of Health Payment

If information technology will make "continuous" relationships between physicians and their patients and families, at some point, we have to question why federal healthcare payment continues to revolve around paying a la carte for physical encounters like physician office visits or hospitalizations. Current Medicare and private payment policy contains inappropriate incentives, not only to maximize provider income by doing more, perhaps, than patients may need to care for them, but, by implication, to wait until a disease progresses far enough to justify more lucrative, high-technology intervention.

Maintenance of health, disease management, advice and counseling—these are not the focus of the current healthcare payment schemes. Furthermore, as we enter an era of increasingly precise genetic prediction, the economy is already laboring to take care of the 5 percent of the population who are sick; how can it possibly finance care for everyone who has some genetic risk of illness?

Rather than continuing to use a transaction-driven (e.g., per visit or per hospital episode) healthcare payment system, the optimal way of paying for health services in an electronically enabled healthcare world would be a relationship-driven payment system (Figure 7.1). Ideally, physicians would be paid a monthly or annual subscription fee for each consumer who signed up to be cared for by the physician. Some of the emerging and controversial concepts in physician practice, like so-called "boutique medicine," where consumers pay a fee to enter a physician's practice, anticipate this subscription model.

The key to the subscription is establishing electronic connectivity between the consumer and the physician he or she has chosen. After electronic connectivity has been established between consumers and providers, maintaining electronic contact with consumers should be far less costly than under a visit-and-telephone-consultation system. Many interactions that required patient visits under the old system could be handled "asynchronously" under the electronic system, with software assistance supported by the physician's office staff.

Many functions, like prescription renewals, transmittal of vital signs, scheduling, and billing, that were handled in person or through telephone interactions could be automated through Internet applications and managed by the physician's or hospital's staff. In addition, someone other than the physician may handle many requests for information.

Subscription fees would cover maintenance of the 24/7 connections, as well as the cost of most services the consumer would use in a year. The fees would be paid to the principal physician by the health plan or federal government, which would be functioning not as a fiscally interested intermediary, but rather as a sponsor of the relationship. The costs of periodic screening both for genetic and cellular abnormalities would be included in the subscription amount.

Hospitalizations and other relatively rare medical interventions would probably be paid separately from the subscription amount. These costs, as well as those of specialists and consultants, would

Figure 7.1: Digital Medicine—Past and Future

PAST	FUTURE
• Event-driven	• Continuous
• Fee-for-service	• Subscription
• Separate records	• Single record
• Payer as intermediary	• Payer as sponsor
• Provider driven	• Customer driven
• "Right stuff"–based clinical decision support	• Science-based clinical decision support

Source: Health Futures, Inc.

probably be incorporated into some type of "per episode of illness" payment to the physician responsible for care for that illness or condition. These per-episode payments would be larger for older consumers or those with complex health problems. In payment jargon, this is sometimes called a "severity-adjusted case rate."

The payment rates with hospitals would probably be negotiated by the health plans or the federal government directly, but the amount and nature of care would continue to be subject to physician control. Physicians should have broad discretion in determining what type of services are provided, but should have an incentive to economize where possible. As with surgical procedures, hospitalizations would carry a substantial consumer cost share, based on ability to pay.

The method of payment should be neutral on the cost of immunizations and immune therapy. The custom fabrication of immunizations or other forms of therapy based on the consumer's genotype would be treated as an "episode of care" like a surgical procedure, but to encourage these preventive measures, the cost should be borne separately by the health plan and be shared modestly with the patient or the physician to encourage them to be used.

Health Policy Issues Raised by Information Technology 167

Substantial consumer cost sharing, graded to income, would be essential to exert a braking influence on procedure costs. Thus, consumers and physicians would have the same incentive to avoid unnecessary care, or care that could be made unnecessary by successful management of identified health risks.

The "intelligent" clinical information system discussed earlier could provide the information base not only to analyze patterns of healthcare spending, but also to determine the most effective methods of care. Analysis of this information across large groups of patients could give to providers at risk for the cost of care the tools and information needed to make intelligent decisions about how to maximize the health of their subscribers. This information was missing in nearly all of the examples where physicians groups attempted to manage "capitated" payment during the 1990s (and went broke doing it).

The principal way that physicians would increase their income is by enrolling more consumers and by minimizing the amount of curative medicine their patients need. They would grow their practices by earning higher consumer satisfaction evaluations and garnering referrals from satisfied customers. These satisfaction scores would be posted on consumer web sites and be available to help guide consumers' choice of physicians. Physicians who do an especially skillful job of organizing their connectivity and support for consumers, particularly responding to consumer questions and managing disease-management protocols, could handle a larger panel of consumers than physicians today.

The more effective physicians are in helping consumers identify and manage their medical risks, the more they earn. To encourage this, physician fees for medical and surgical procedures should be paid out of the per-episode-of-care amount, creating incentives for physicians to work with their consumers to minimize the need for these procedures.

Under a subscription system, physicians who continued relying on patient visits and telephone interactions would have higher overhead and not be able to "scale up" effectively to handle larger groups of consumers/subscribers. Computer technology and effective support staffing could markedly improve physician productivity as well as result in better health outcomes for subscribers.

Will Changing the Financial Incentives Really Control the Cost of Care?

We must begin thinking as a society about how to manage a potential quantum increase in health expenses. This expense increase would occur with a constant population that was not aging, given the technological advances that have been discussed. Add to this technological transformation an expanding population and the impending retirement of a 76-million-person cohort of baby boomers (whose oldest members are 57 in 2003), and one has all the necessary ingredients for fiscal catastrophe.

A significant future rise in health costs is inevitable. How the responsibility for paying for that rise is distributed among the various responsible parties is the essential societal debate.[10] Whether an objective social and political dialog can take place about how to apportion future health cost risks is complicated by the costly myth of "entitlement without responsibility" that continues to pervade the American political system.

The emerging predictive tools and expensive remedies for disease beg the question of how much longer this can remain a tenable way of thinking about health financing. The concept of identifiable genetic disease risk and the (slowly) emerging capability to manage those risks will give our society powerful new tools to improve the quality of our lives.

In the face of these emerging technologies, continuing to view healthcare as something to which consumers are simply entitled, to be paid for with someone else's money, under economic incentives that encourage physicians to maximize their income by doing more, is irresponsible social policy. Finding a humane and responsible balance of risk and responsibility for health and health cost is the most unpleasant but necessary piece of health policy on the national horizon.

NOTES

1. Princeton Survey Research Associates. 1999. "Medical Privacy and Confidentiality Survey: Summary and Overview." [Online information; retrieved 12/05/02.] http://www.chcf.org/topics/view.cfm?itemID=12500.

2. Goldman, J. 1998. "Protecting Privacy to Improve Health Care." *Health Affairs* 17 (6): 47–60.

3. Westin, A. 2001. *Privacy and American Business,* October.

4. Westin, A. 2001. Personal communication, October.

5. Ibid.

6. Kongstvedt, P., and H. Shaman. 2000. *Managed Care Measures: Result of the 1999 Benchmarking Study.* Washington, DC: Ernst & Young.

7. Cunningham, R. 2000. "Old Before Its Time: HIPAA and E-Health Policy." *Health Affairs* 19 (6): 231–38.

8. Goldsmith, J. 1992. "The Reshaping of Healthcare." *Healthcare Forum Journal* 35 (3): 18–22, 25–27.

9. Goldsmith, J., D. Blumenthal, and W. Rishel. 2003. "Federal Health Information Policy: A Case of Arrested Development." *Health Affairs* 22 (4): 45–55.

10. Goldsmith, J. 2003. "Road to Reform: Interview with Oregon's John Kitzhaber." *Health Affairs* 22 (1): 114–24.

CHAPTER 8

Making an Effective Digital Transformation

THIS BOOK HAS outlined how information technology is transforming our troubled health system. By the time this transformation is completed, our health system will be wired (as well as wireless), more intelligent, and much more responsive to both consumers and caregivers. Would that such a system existed today.

Nevertheless, those who are interested in having such a system in the near future must be sobered by the difficulty for the health system to achieve real change. There are many reasons why healthcare has lagged as much as 20 years behind other sectors of the economy in taking up and using IT's powerful toolbox. Some of these reasons are excusable, but many are not. If this lag is to end the behavior of the health system's actors—physicians, managers, trustees, directors, investors, and vendors of IT products—must change.

Although the complexity of healthcare itself is partly responsible for the lag in application of IT, the weakness of institutional leadership and followership and the quality of IT products themselves must take their share of the blame as well. Despite Moore's Law and the plummeting cost of hardware, IT in healthcare is still very expensive. This is explained by a corollary proposition, first made by

Nathan Myrvold, the former chief technology officer for Microsoft, who once said, "Software is a gas. It expands to fill available storage space."

Software development has not kept pace with hardware advances because it is exceptionally difficult to discipline and manage. It has been easier for software firms to grow through acquisition and patch together interfaces than to fundamentally reexamine how their tools can be used to make healthcare better. Making investments in expensive, unstable, and complex products has engendered appropriate caution and, in some quarters, cynicism among healthcare executives and physicians about whether the promised benefits of IT innovation can ever be achieved.

Healthcare managers have been guilty, however, of assuming that simply purchasing and installing clinical software is enough to achieve real transformation. The reality is that transformation of care processes and relationships must be an explicit objective of the organization, with board, executive management, and clinical leadership all committed to making their contribution to achieving that transformation.

Clinical software is the means to that end. Transformation is not a task that can be delegated to the vendor, because neither the vendor nor the chief information officer who manages the vendor relationship has enough power to change how care is actually rendered in healthcare organizations.

PHYSICIAN ACCEPTANCE: A SIGNIFICANT HURDLE TO ADOPTION

Physicians pose a particular challenge in implementing new clinical information solutions. Many physicians still practice solo or in small groups. Thus, their businesses have little leverage of scale and are thinly capitalized and vulnerable. Conservatism and risk aversion are understandable in this setting. Physicians also, legitimately, have high functional hurdles. Technologies need to solve problems, and if they do not, physicians literally have no time for them.

Physicians are not, as I have earlier argued, allergic to technology. They embrace the technologies that help them. However, physicians are exceptionally conservative as actors in the health system. Many have a small-business mentality and practice outside the sphere of the hospitals they use. Even in large groups and health systems, physicians tend to behave not as institutional citizens, but as free agents. They are often depressingly resistant both to leadership by their peers and to change itself.

Although many profess to feel powerless, physicians tend to exercise veto power over initiatives in hospitals and physician organizations where they feel their personal interests are compromised, even if broader benefits can be achieved by cooperating. This is why physician leadership is a vital component of an effective digital transformation. Mobilizing a cadre of physician supporters is the essential ingredient in any successful clinical transformation. Toward this end, many healthcare organizations are appointing chief medical informatics officers or their equivalents to provide a focus and rallying point for physician involvement in healthcare transformation. It is far easier for physicians to be convinced by colleagues than by lay managers of the need for change. Physicians are likely to be the most persuasive change agents among their own professional colleagues and can lead change with the rest of the clinical team.

Unless physicians accept the need to change workflow and clinical processes and for improved communications within the clinical team, those changes simply will not occur. Moreover, physician skepticism about the need for change will infect the rest of the clinical team and engender resistance by nursing personnel and others on whom physicians depend for support. This is why soliciting physician input into IT implementation is essential early and continuously through the process.

Physicians are also going to need to accept hospital help with digitizing their clinical operations in their offices and harmonizing them with the hospitals' clinical systems. This is likely to be a tall order in many places, where an unfortunate legacy of the 1990s has been heightened mistrust between physicians and hospital managers.

In the 1980s and early 1990s, physicians actively resisted any effort by the hospital to reach out to the physician's office with connectivity strategies, such as remote order entry and retrieval of test results. Many physicians felt that hospitals would be tracking their clinical activities and using the information they generated to control physician behavior. Physicians feared information system linkages to the hospital would be used to profile physicians who practiced "expensive" medicine and enable the hospital to practice so-called "economic credentialing" (e.g., excluding those whose orders or admitting patterns caused the hospital to lose money).

New approaches may be needed to bring hospital and physician systems together. One interesting approach was devised by the Concord (NH) Hospital. Rather than converting hospital records first, it encouraged all of the physicians in the community to standardize their office clinical systems on a common platform. Then the hospital made it possible for physicians to connect to and edit their office records through dial-up connections inside the hospital, postponing the conversion of the hospital's record systems until physicians had become "addicted" to a more convenient electronic practice styles.

Suspicion of hospital motives linger, and these must be alleviated if a truly safe patient care environment is to be created. Just as hospitals must convince patients and their families that their electronic clinical records will be protected and used judiciously and only by those who need to be involved directly in the care process, so too must hospitals convince physicians that an integrated record platform will be used in a way that preserves the privacy and integrity of the physician's practice. To do so is not technically complex. The key ingredient is trust and consistent, fair behavior by hospital managers.

In the past two years, I have noticed a sea change in physician attitudes toward their hospitals' IT strategy. Physicians in many parts of the country have ceased resisting IT innovation and have begun aggressively urging hospitals to convert to electronic medical records, physician order entry, and "practice anywhere" wireless IT tools. Physicians are coming to realize that IT can make it much more convenient to practice medicine and are urging hospitals to push more capabilities for managing the patient care process out to their offices or, through wireless technology, to their Palms or PDAs. If physicians make it clear to hospitals that they need to make it easier for them to practice medicine, hospital managers and boards will respond.

When physicians talk, hospital boards and managers listen. All too often, physicians have used their power to stop the hospital from doing things to change the status quo. However, with IT innovation, physicians have the opportunity to speed the transformation of the hospital's clinical and financial information systems to make the hospital easier to use.

HOSPITALS AT THE IT CROSSROADS: BALANCING COMPETING PRIORITIES

Those who manage and govern the nation's almost 5,000 community hospitals have faced difficulties in the late 1990s and early 2000s. The cumulative impact of managed care payment reductions and Medicare spending caps from the Balanced Budget Act of 1997 decimated hospital operating margins and cash flows. Hospital credit deteriorated, and many hospitals responded by reducing staff and curtailing capital spending.

At the same time, stress and poorly organized workflow continued driving away skilled hospital workers. As of this writing, many hospitals have critical shortages of nurses, pharmacists, radiology technicians, and a host of other skilled professional workers. Many hospital executives have not connected the present scarcity of skilled workers to the systemic problem of a stressful and desolating work environment.

Hospital professionals enter the field to help other people, to take care of the sick and dying. They do not enter the field to drown in a sea of paperwork, boring meetings, and unreturned telephone calls. Although other factors, such as a perception of a loss of control over their work environment and lack of respect by physicians and management, certainly play a role, the catastrophic state of information systems in hospitals has contributed materially to the stress and lack of work satisfaction of the hospital workforce.

Information technology is expensive. As hospital capital budgets have been squeezed, spending on IT has been forced to compete with the hospital's traditional construction and major equipment needs for limited dollars. In the general economy, IT accounts for 40 percent or more of all capital spending. Traditionally, in hospitals, the ratio has been far lower—10 to 20 percent is more typical. The result has been paradoxical: beautiful buildings with state-of-the-art clinical technology are supported by third-world IT that frustrates and demoralizes the hospital workforce.

The good news is that IT will become more affordable in future years. This is not only because of increasing competition among IT vendors, but also because the Internet will make it possible for many complex applications, including electronic medical records, to be hosted remotely and paid for as part of the operations budget. After installation, which will remain a capital expense, much of the complexity and cost of operation will be borne by the vendor or an outsourcing partner and managed much more efficiently in a central location. Internet connectivity is also going to make complex healthcare computing more accessible to smaller hospitals and physician clinic settings.

THE CHALLENGE OF MANAGING IT IN HOSPITALS

Hospital managers did not, as a rule, receive instruction in their graduate educations about IT. Information technology is like Roman Polanski's *Chinatown* to many hospital CEOs—a dangerous place where people speak a foreign tongue and you never figure out what's going on before something horrible happens to you. Many CEOs delay making IT investments because they simply do not feel comfortable with the choices they are presented. (CEOs interested in learning more about IT strategy should read John Glaser's useful and readable book *The Strategic Application of IT in Health Care Organizations*, Second Edition, San Francisco: Jossey Bass, 2002.)

The hospital's information professionals are stretched inhumanly thin repairing and renovating the hospital's legacy systems. Furthermore, they are politically hamstrung by the hospital's fragmented department structure. They are often the only "lobby" in the hospital's management structure for standardization and ease of information flow between departments. No wonder the turnover of hospital chief information officers is so high and that there are so many vacancies in technical positions in hospital IT.

IS OUTSOURCING IT AN OPTION?

One major management decision boards and executives face in the coming years is whether to continue managing IT in house or to contract with outside firms to manage it. Business process outsourcing (as opposed to outsourcing food service, for example) is a reliable means that high-technology industries have used to achieve rapid change in manufacturing, supplier, and customer relationships.[1]

Business process outsourcing is new to healthcare, but it is eventually going to be a hundred-billion-dollar business. The business office, including billing and collections, human resources, and materials management are also major functions amenable to outsourcing solutions. Under the right circumstances, and with the right partner, outsourcing IT management provides management both the control of and the distance from the minutiae that are needed to effect meaningful change. For those executives who question the depth and capabilities of their in-house IT operations, outsourcing the management of clinical and business systems is a real option.

Managing the contract is a complex challenge. One does not cease employing in-house IT managers in an outsourcing mode. Rather, the IT managers are there to manage the contract and the relationship with the vendor and to provide the local knowledge and "political" wisdom and judgment to implement new IT solutions. The contract should also specify functional and economic "end points" that the vendor is expected to achieve, and it should provide financial incentives for achieving them, as well as penalties for failing to achieve them. Outsourcing does not mean surrendering accountability for achieving a more efficient, safer hospital. It is, fundamentally, a partnership through which the hospital acquires skills, knowledge, and personnel from outside the organization to accomplish a complex task.

MANAGING THE VENDORS

During the past 20 years, healthcare executives have been ill served by the vendors of IT to their field. Information technology vendors have consistently misrepresented their current capabilities to impress investor analysts and institutional investors who buy or recommend their stock. Vendors often demonstrate products at professional meetings that exist only on PowerPoint slides, with real code and function to follow. Gullible hospital executives who want to be on the cutting edge, but who have not done enough homework to understand how mature a technology is or whether a vendor can actually deliver when they saw in the PowerPoint slides, feel ill-used. Hospital and health system executives need to assume a portion of the blame for what has been historically a very troubled relationship.

There's a remedy for this dance of disappointment. Instead of signing speculative contracts based on unproven technology, hospital executives should simply say, "Take me to a facility where your product is actually running." Surely this is not too much to ask before making a multimillion-dollar capital spending decision. When the management team arrives at the demonstration site, its members should fan out into the patient floors, clinics, and operating suites and start asking the users, including patients, nursing staff, and physicians, how well the product is working. The hospital's IT staff should be queried on the project's schedule and costs and the support relationship they experienced with the vendor. If the product cannot run without the vendor's technical and marketing staffs nervously hovering about, the team should fly home and begin looking elsewhere for IT solutions.

This is not to say that hospitals should not be willing to experiment with vendors and serve as alpha test sites for new technologies. The willingness to take some risks to explore promising applications is vital if the field is to advance technically. Managers should simply enter into alpha-type relationships with eyes open, knowing that they are engaged in an experiment, not the installation of a proven product. The project should be tested in a venturesome, well-managed corner of the hospital or system and ramped up rapidly in the rest of the organization if it works.

As a general rule, hospitals should pay vendors based on project completion milestones, with both incentives for rapid and effective installation and penalties for missed deadlines and budgets. If savings in reduced staff are to be achieved, project completion payments should be conditioned upon actually achieving the savings.

Managing the change process in the hospital's clinical and support departments is not something that can be delegated to the vendor. Being willing to provide leadership and to not tolerate bureaucratic excuses and political gamesmanship from inside the organization is critical to ensuring a timely and effective conversion.

Hospital executives must also be willing to learn the language. They must shed the reluctance to expose themselves to the complexities of IT and delve into this field. Becoming IT literate and developing a greater sense of self-confidence in making IT investments is going to be essential if hospital management is prevail in the coming decades. This is not to suggest that one dispenses with the advice and support of one's CIO or IT staff. Rather, the dialog with them must move to a higher level.

Managing and incorporating IT into the hospital is going to be a central strategic challenge for hospital managers for the next 20 years. Hospitals have historically had great difficulty implementing change of any sort. The risk/reward relationship for innovation in hospital management has been adverse to the innovators. Unless hospital and health system managers make the transformation in clinical and management process at the heart of adopting new IT their number one or number two priority, it simply is not going to happen.

THE BOARD'S IT CHALLENGE

For boards, the largest challenge may be to redefine their roles to force more accountability both for resource use and for patient safety. As argued earlier, IT by itself is not going to make hospitals or other healthcare organizations safer or better places in which to work. This is a task for leadership, and leadership begins at the board level. Board members in the largely not-for-profit hospital system hold assets in trust for the benefit of the whole community. Maximizing that benefit has been an elusive goal for many hospital boards.

Earlier, it was suggested that the reason why enterprise computing in healthcare has been such a challenge is that, in reality, many healthcare organizations are not enterprises at all. This is because individual professions or professionals have retained the power to veto or delay important organizational changes that could benefit patients and the institution as a whole.

A major reason for this is reticence by the board to make choices and to support their managers when they do so. Decisions that may seem both sensible and dispassionate at the board level have direct economic effects on incomes, employment, and working conditions of health professionals, particularly physicians, who often use the hospital's capital at no personal risk to generate substantial personal incomes for themselves.

It has been suggested that an effective information system is like a nervous system. A central nervous system is, among other things, a powerful tool for making and implementing decisions on behalf of the whole organism (not its individual limbs or organs). To take advantage of having a central nervous system, however, it is important to have a spine.[2]

A major reason why many hospitals and health systems behave more like amoebae than higher organisms is because of weak governance. Hospital boards must be more willing than in the past to function as the spine of their organizations. Separating strong from weak claims on institutional resources and being less tolerant of excuses for institutional practices that expose patients to unacceptable risks are two important things boards can do to safeguard their community's trust.

The balancing of hospital capital-spending priorities has been one of the traditional roles of the hospital board. Constructing buildings is one of the exciting things hospital boards have traditionally done. There is something reassuringly concrete about a new building, and you can name it after someone. Alternatively, a hospital information system is not visible (wiring never is). To my knowledge, no one has ever named an information system after a major donor.

Boards must reexamine their spending priorities and decide how important it is to have a humane, responsive clinical care system. Reducing medication errors, improving communication between physicians and the care system, improving patient safety, and more efficiently charging for and collecting for a hospital's services will require increased, and more intelligent, investment in IT. In some cases, this will mean postponing construction projects. In other cases, hospital managers will discover that the reason they have capacity problems in the first place is because IT does not support efficient scheduling, results reporting, and care coordination.[3]

Purchasing and installing new IT is expensive and disruptive of established routines. Some of those routines need disrupting, as they do not support safe and effective patient care. Hospital boards must be prepared to be a little less patient and tolerant of excuses that serve to delay the wiring of their institutions. Electronic clinical and financial systems will bring greater discipline and focus to patient care decisions. Boards and managers need to hasten an era of greater accountability for decisions that affect patients' lives. After all, the lives they save could be their own.

THE NEED FOR INVESTORS TO BE PATIENT

A major lesson from the Internet health bubble was how long it takes for healthcare institutions and practitioners to adopt and use new IT tools. Venture firms, bankers, pension fund and mutual fund managers, and individual investors seemed to be playing on 78 rpm while the customer was listening on 33 rpm. The tragedy of e-health was that these radically different expectation sets were never harmonized. One wonders whether those who invest in and influence capital markets learned the right lessons from the e-health debacle.

Most e-health firms were funded by venture capital firms whose managers and investors expected 30 percent per year compounded annual returns on their capital and a public market for their investments to materialize within three years. Given the superheated stock market in the late 1990s, it was actually possible to field a new company and take it public within 18 months (with "revenues," but often no earnings). This was a marvelous, if unreal, economic environment for venture capitalists, who were enabled in their search for a quick exit by breathless and starry-eyed investors.

Nothing meaningful in healthcare happens in three years' time. Federal regulatory approvals impose seven- to ten-year lead times on new discoveries in biotechnology and conventional pharmaceutical research. For medical devices, approval times are shorter, although not dramatically so. Closer to our subject, complex software development in healthcare often takes five years or more from the gleam in the software architect's eye to a finished, debugged, and installed product. Given capital spending cycles in hospitals and health plans, the process of contracting for new IT applications, and the agony of installation, it may be five to seven years between the time that a new technology surfaces and its actual realization by users.[4]

It is not that the market opportunity is not there, either. Hospitals and health systems could be spending as much as $30 billion a year by the end of the decade on IT. To develop the software and supporting infrastructure for the important applications discussed in this book will require tens of billions of dollars in investment. The challenge for investors is simply that this field is unfolding at what seems like a glacial pace, given the metabolism of large, complex health enterprises and markets.

Gartner, the premier IT consultanting firm, has a marvelous construct to explain the impact of exaggerated expectations in IT. It is called the "hype cycle" (Figure 8.1). In our technologically obsessed society, it is almost inevitable that we overestimate the short-run impact and market significance of new technologies when they are introduced (in a wave of hype). There follows a similarly inevitable disillusionment when one realizes that the technologies are not "finished" and need refinement to be truly useful.

In healthcare IT, the time required for a technology to survive the plunge into disillusionment and morph into something indispensable may be three to five years or more. In biotechnology and genomics, it may take seven to ten years or more.

Not all technologies survive the plunge. If the disillusionment is pervasive enough, a technology becomes unloved and unfinanceable. No one is willing to take the risk. However, many of the technologies that do survive go on to become indispensable. The key to becoming indispensable is for vendors and their engineering and marketing staffs to develop strong feedback loops with their customers and users and rewrite and rescope their products until they solve a real problem or meet a real need. This is difficult because

Figure 8.1: Hype Cycle for Healthcare Provider Technologies, 2003

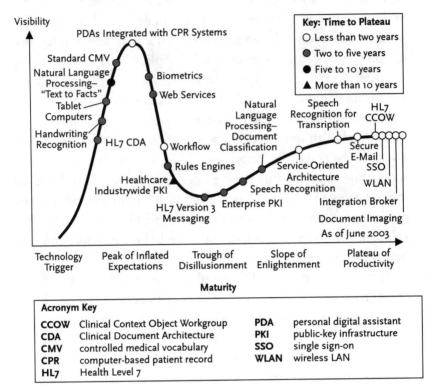

Source: Gartner Research. © 2003 Gartner, Inc. and/or Its Affiliates. All Rights Reserved.

engineers tend to be driven by a cultural value of "Isn't it cool that we can do this?" Customers tend to be more focused: "Cool does not mean useful. Does this solve a real problem for us?"

Information technology tools almost never work correctly the first time they are used. One only truly learns to use IT by fiddling with it and modifying it until it meets one's needs. Having the patience to recognize the ultimate value of a technology and to tolerate the fiddling is necessary to make it truly useful. Successful IT companies will foster this collaborative searching for functions that really make a difference. Successful investors will understand that this process requires patience and confidence in the managers and scientists they support.

All of this suggests an urgent need by venture investors and the equity markets to revise their expectations of the pace and magnitude of capital returns in IT. Healthcare applications require "warm" money—returns in the high teens and time frames of seven to ten years and the patience to retest assumptions about what actually works in the field. Although the development of enterprise clinical and financial software in healthcare seem to be consolidating into firms whose original business was manufacturing medical equipment (GE, Philips, Siemens, etc.), the field remains ripe for start-up firms with bright ideas and unconventional approaches.

MAKING IT HAPPEN

Americans have a schizophrenic attitude toward technological progress, perhaps best depicted in the marvelous sorcerer's apprentice sequence from Walt Disney's *Fantasia.* On the one hand, technology is magic and can make dreams reality. On the other hand, technology changes lives in ways one cannot anticipate or control. Technology has a funny way of morphing into an end in itself unless it is wielded and controlled by a strong, purposeful hand.

In the final analysis, there is no good excuse for healthcare applications of IT lagging 20 years or more behind the adoption rate in other industries. Americans (and people in other countries as well) have paid the price for this lag in absurd paperwork burdens, excessive administrative costs, delayed or unresponsive decision making, burned-out caregivers and managers, a consumer-unresponsive and unfriendly healthcare experience, and an unacceptably high risk of adverse events. Emerging information technologies can change all these things with the right combination of patience, financing, and intolerance of excuses and poor performance.

The key to achieving a more intelligent, responsive, and safer health system is to raise collective expectations of how the health system performs. All of us, in our roles as consumers, practitioners, managers, trustees, capital funders, and policymakers, can influence the pace of transformation. The technology by itself is not enough. Thoughtful application of these powerful new tools can create a better healthcare experience and improved health. It will not simply happen by itself.

NOTES

1. Goldman, S., and C. Graham, eds. 1999. *Agility in Healthcare: Strategies for Mastering Turbulent Markets*. San Francisco: Jossey-Bass.

2. Newcomer, L., executive vice president, Vivuis; former chief medical officer, United HealthGroup. Personal communication, 2002.

3. Goldsmith, J. 2002. "The Capital Conundrum. Balancing Needs Under Pressure." *Trustee* 55 (9): 10–13.

4. Glaser, J., vice president and CIO, Partners HealthCare. Personal communication, 2001.

Index

187

Health-Market, 134
Health payment transactions, 156
Health plans: Consumer Choice, 126; consumer safety and, 128; customers, 125–27; defined-benefit *vs.* defined contribution, 136; digitizing, 140–41; disease management and, 131; e-commerce and, 120; economic incentives of, 139, 146; efficient, 120; financial recovery of, 117; genetic prediction and, 159–60; Internet and, 118; IT and, 119; management of, 124; medical errors and, 128; paper and, 120–22; privacy and, 160; quality maps of, 128; reform, 141; reprogramming, 122; standardization of, 162–63; switching, 147, 160; telephone and, 118–19; virtual, 134
Health reform, 108
Health risks: AI and, 10–11; consumers and, 95; diagnosing, 9–10
Health services: electronic payment of, 141; modernizing, 7–8
Health software, 61–64
Health spending, 96
Health systems, 12; genetics and, 19; market value of, 1
Heart attack damage, 22
Heart disease, genetics and, 14
Heart rhythms: Medtronic and, 26; monitoring, 25
HELP, 34
HER-2, 17
Herceptin, 17
Hertz, 36
HHS. *See* Department of Health and Human Services, U.S.
Hill-Burton, 163
HIPAA. *See* Health Insurance Portability and Accountability Act of 1996
Hippocrates, 96
HIV. *See* Human immunodeficiency virus
HMO claims, 119
Hospitalization: payment of, 166–67; risks of, 63

Hospital-physician information boundary, 50, 85–88
Hospital(s): allocation, 50; billing, 48; boards, 180–82; CEOs, 177; clinical records, 128, 174; competition in, 50; computing, 48–52; connecting, 55–60; cost of HIPAA for, 157–58; credit, 175; education, 179; health insurance and, 140–41; health software, 61–64; heart, 50; as information source, 85–86; IT, 48; IT management, 176–77; IT spending, 176; management, 176, 179–80; medical records and, 164; new technologies in, 47; not-for-profit, 87, 164; occupancy, 25–26; outsourcing, 59–60; payment rates with, 167; PHRs and, 58; politics, 51; priorities of, 175–76; professionals, 176; quality standards, 129; revenues, 47; selection, 96, 102; shared services at, 62; staffing shortages, 175; vendor relationships, 48; versus private practice, 85–86; wireless technology in, 41
Housekeeping, 59
Humana, 118–19; IT investment of, 142
Human engineering, 40
Human Genome Project, 15
Human immunodeficiency virus (HIV), 16; therapy, 17–18
Human judgment, 24
Human resources: outsourcing, 60, 177
Human waste, 101
Huntington's disease, 15
Hype cycle, 183
Hypertension, 130; management, 79

IBM, 62
ICU. *See* Intensive care unit
IDX, 34
Image recognition software, 24
Imaging technologies, 10, 11; molecular, 18; noninvasive, 47
Immune response, 18
Immunizations, 167
Implantable devices, 26

Infection(s): genomics and, 16; hospital-borne, 63, 128; rates, 128; spinal cord, 100

Information: availability of, 100; flow, 101; prescription, 78; processing, 60; resource, 107–8; standardization, 121–22; XML and, 9

Information technology (IT), 1; adoption, 172–75, 185; application of, 185–86; benefits of, 11, 74–76; benefit-to-cost ratio of, 64; care coordination, 181; clinical, 87; complexity of, 61; for consumers, 112; contracts, 178; costs, 12, 41, 119, 176; cost savings of, 11; cycles, 183; demonstration, 179; development, 34–35; disruptions, 182; education, 179–80; expectations, 183–85; expenditures, 2; failures, 119; in group practices, 72; health plans and, 118, 119, 127; in hospitals, 48; improvements in, 8; incorporating, 180; innovation, 175; international, 73–74; investment, 63–64, 142; lag, 7–8, 171; management, 30, 176–77, 177–78; medical errors and, 130; medical practice and, 72–73; outsourcing, 177–78; patience with, 184–85; payment for, 163–64; physician resistance to, 70; privacy and, 153; promise of, 88; reorganization and, 41; results reporting, 181; scheduling, 181; slow adoption of, 54; spending, 183; staff, 180; subscribing to, 63; trust in, 174; vendors, 54, 62, 178

Informed Choice, 132–33

Institute of Medicine (IOM), 6

Insurance: risk evaluation, 146; verification, 120, 121; See also Health insurance

Intel, 22

Intelligent agents, 110

Intensive care unit (ICU): APACHE and, 34; remote monitoring in, 25; staffing of, 129

Intermountain Health Care, 31; 3M Corporation and, 33

Internal Revenue Code, 87

Internet, 28–31; advent of, 8; ASP and, 8–9; backlash, 108; billing and, 57; chronic care and, 132; connectivity, 176; consumerism and, 101–3; consumers and, 56, 94; digital imaging and, 24; disease management and, 131; effects of, 30–31; frustration, 107; health bubble, 182; health information on, 7; health plans and, 142; HIPAA and, 158–59; importance of, 12; information flow on, 101; mass customization, 133; medical records and, 80; network computing and, 55–56; outsourcing and, 57, 60; peer connections on, 82; personal health records and, 57–58; scheduling and, 57; second opinion consultations on, 80; start-up companies, 58; usage, 29, 102; XML and, 9

Internet service provider (ISP), 159

Interoperating, 33

Intranets, 56; digital imaging and, 10

Inurement of benefit, 87

Investors, 182–85

IOM. See Institute of Medicine

ISDN, 75

ISP. See Internet service provider

IT. See Information technology

Jackson Hole Group, 126

Jefferson, Thomas, 138

Jellyfish, 53

Johns Hopkins University: medical knowledge and, 110; Partners Health System and, 80

Joint Commission of Accreditation of Healthcare Organizations, 162

Kassebaum-Kennedy Act. See Health Insurance Portability and Accountability Act of 1996

Keypad, 39

Kidnapping, 103

Kleinke, J. D., 52

Knaus, William, 34

Knowledge archive, 84
knowledge-based professions, 106
Knowledge pathway, 96–98
Knowledgeware, 162

Laparascope, 27
Lasers: diffraction patterns of, 20; flow
    cytometry and, 20
Laundry, 59
Law enforcement agencies, 148
Leadership, 55; outsourcing and, 179
Leapfrog Group, 129
Legal barriers, 86–87
Lehigh University, 63
Lesions: detection of, 24; diagnosis of, 22
Lewis, Michael, 105–6
Lobbying organizations, 157
Lotus Notes, 82
Luddites, 70
Luminos, 134
Lupus, 107

MacLean, Norman, 99–100
MacNealy, Scott, 149
Magnetic pulse, 20
Magnetic resonance imaging (MRI), 10;
    Internet and, 24; modifications to,
    21–22
Magnetic resonance spectroscopy, 22
Malpractice, 162
Mammograms, machine-read, 24
Managed care: adoption of, 68; assump-
    tions of, 117; consumer contributions
    in, 138; contracts, 68; criticism of,
    67; failures, 117; growth of, 118–19;
    payment reductions, 175; reform,
    123–25, 126
Marketing, search engines and, 111
Market solutions, 165
Massachusetts General, 80
Mass customization, 133
Mass media, 98
Materials management: outsourcing, 60,
    177
Mayo Clinic, 82; consumer health
    information, 111; medical knowledge
    and, 110

McDonald, Clem, 56
Medicaid, 145
Medical device approvals, 182–83
Medical education sessions, 69
Medical encounter information, 59
Medical errors, 6; IT and, 11, 55; reporting,
    128, 162–63; variation of, 130
Medical information: broadband connec-
    tivity and, 13; pre-digital, 13; privacy
    of, 156; protection of, 146; security
    of, 156
Medical journals, 83; digitized, 6
Medical knowledge, 93; accessibility of,
    108; access to, 112–14; acquiring,
    96–97; digital, 6; evolution of, 39;
    future of, 107–8; IT and, 88; new,
    5–6, 37; physicians and, 106; time
    lag of, 98; transmitting, 81; trusted
    sources of, 110
Medical management, 120; Internet and,
    124–25
Medical paternalism, 109
Medical practice, 72–73
Medical records: automating, 85–86;
    connectivity to, 164; departmental,
    51; differing systems of, 4; digitizing,
    87–88, 153; electronic versus paper,
    13–14; genetic information in, 10;
    Internet and, 80; law enforcement
    agencies and, 148; paper, 2–3, 4,
    153; physician, 4, 50; privacy of,
    153; sharing, 4; See also Electronic
    medical records
Medical vocabulary, 39; controlled, 161
Medicare, 145, 155; chronic disease and, 130;
    claims, 163; CMS and, 129; disease
    management and, 131; genetic
    prediction and, 160; HIPAA and,
    161; outlays, 158; payment freeze of,
    123; payment policy, 165; regulations,
    86–87; spending caps, 175
Medication: errors, 128, 181; genetically
    customized, 18; reminders, 28
MEDLINE, 5, 83; citations in, 107
Medscape, 83
Medtronic, 26; clinical information
    systems and, 38

About the Author

JEFF GOLDSMITH is president of Health Futures, Inc., and associate professor of medical education in the College of Medicine at the University of Virginia. He has taught health policy and management at the University of Chicago Graduate School of Business, the Wharton School at the University of Pennsylvania, and other leading universities. Mr. Goldsmith received his doctorate in sociology from the University of Chicago in 1973. He worked for the governor of Illinois as a policy analyst and the dean of the Pritzker School of Medicine at the University of Chicago, where he was responsible for planning and government affairs for the Medical Center.

Mr. Goldsmith is a member of the board of directors of the Cerner Corporation, a healthcare informatics firm, and Essent Healthcare, an investor-owned hospital management company, and he is a member of the board of advisors of the Burrill Life Sciences Capital Fund, which invests in biotechnology innovation. He is also an advisor to Cain Brothers, an investment banking firm that works exclusively in healthcare.

Mr. Goldsmith's principal activity is forecasting technological and economic trends in the health system. He has consulted widely for firms spanning the health system spectrum, including hospital systems, health plans, medical device and product firms, pharmaceutical companies, and multispecialty physician groups. He lives at Ricochet Farm outside Charlottesville, Virginia.